Mine is a story of family and faith, of deep conviction, of hope, of pitting the ravages of cancer against the saving grace of cultivating a healthy body and strong spirit.

The Face of a Miracle

The Face of a Miracle

A Mother, a Son, and the Journey of Life and Faith That Lies in All of Us

Michaelsampson

JODI SAMPSON

Jodi Samps

Proceeds from the sale of this book will go to Pediatric Brain Tumor Research at MassGeneral Hospital for children

TATE PUBLISHING
AND ENTERPRISES, LLC

Author's Note

This is a work of non-fiction. I have rendered the events truthful and honest just as I have recalled them. Many names have been changed to protect individual's privacy. While conversations are depicted in this book, they are my personal recollection, and are not exact word-for word reenactments. They are told for the reader to understand my feelings and my view of what happened at that time.

All Scriptures are taken from:
The Catholic Study Bible
2nd addition New American Bible

The opinions expressed by the author are not necessarily those of Tate Publishing, LLC.

Published by Tate Publishing & Enterprises, LLC
127 E. Trade Center Terrace | Mustang, Oklahoma 73064 USA
1.888.361.9473 | www.tatepublishing.com

Tate Publishing is committed to excellence in the publishing industry. The company reflects the philosophy established by the founders, based on Psalm 68:11,
"The Lord gave the word and great was the company of those who published it."

Published in the United States of America

ISBN: 978-1-68142-278-7
1. Biography & Autobiography / Personal Memoirs
2. Family & Relationships / Parenting / Motherhood
15.09.09

This book is dedicated to Jesus Christ, my Lord and Savior

Mark, my husband
Thank you for your support of our family
through the journey of life.
I counted on your calmness, focus and strength to carry us daily.
Thank you for your love and support of this book and me.

Jordan and Kaitlin, my children
Thank you for your help and guidance with writing
this book. You have enriched my life more than
words can say. I enjoy all there is about
Your individuality and treasure you daily.

Lori Brooks Barish, friend and Editor
Thank you so much for all your time and
talent dedicated to this book. You
Were there at the very beginning typing away at my hand
written scribbling, Always positive and encouraging and making
sense of my writing. This book would not be possible without you.

To All my Family, friends, doctors, nurses, teachers
There are to many people who have helped Michael and my
family to name. You know who you are and my family is
forever grateful for your caring and dedication to all of us

To My Son, Michael
You are the light of my life! Your smile and personality light up
My world! You are a daily inspiration and constant
Reminder of God's infinite love. Your
are strong, brave and the most
Resilient child I know. I thank God for
you every day and love you
With all my heart.

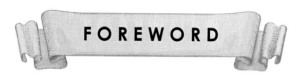

FOREWORD

This is a remarkable, deeply personal, unvarnished portrait of a family's struggles with cancer. We learn how a mother and her family negotiate the despair of a dismal prognosis for their young son diagnosed with an aggressive brain tumor and learn to navigate years of difficult therapy and constant disruptions to the busy routines of a growing family. It is a story about strength and perseverance born of faith, hope and the unselfish kindness of a devoted community of friends who support the Sampson family through their son's long illness and rally behind the author when she must contend with her own devastating illness. This is a brave account of hardships met, of compassion reciprocated and optimism tempered by the recognition that the journey after treatment ends is sometimes just as challenging as the harsh rigors of cancer therapy that mark its beginning.

Dave Ebb, MDPediatric Oncologist
MassGeneral Hospital for Children

CONTENTS

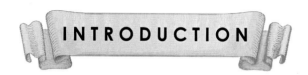

INTRODUCTION

THE DREAM. WE ALL HAVE so many, but the one dream—the dream of our future, our lives—is the big one. As a child, I can remember incessantly playing house. I carefully got my dolls "off to school" and back home for "snacks" then tucked safely into bed, day after day, night after night. As far back as I can remember, I wanted to be a mom. I had other interests too, both domestic; I loved to sew and create things. Perhaps being brought up with *The Brady Bunch* and *The Partridge Family* on television influenced my life more than I knew. The dream of a big, happy family carried me through childhood and into young adulthood.

And I had the dream—for a while. The supportive husband. The big house. Two girls and a boy, conceived after a bit of pregnancy struggles. But we managed it.

Yes, for a while I had the dream.

But just one solemn talk with a doctor changed it all. The perfect child wasn't perfect anymore.

My perfect child, and our perfect life, all came crashing down.

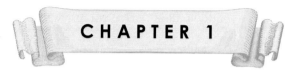

CHAPTER 1

The Dream

I GREW UP IN THE 70s in what would be considered a very typical house in Winthrop, Massachusetts. Winthrop is a small community on the water overlooking Boston Harbor. Houses are like clusters of grapes, and everyone knows everyone. Growing up there, not much went unnoticed. You might say it was very similar to *Mayberry RFD*.

Winthrop was a great place to grow up: a beach around the corner, a great neighborhood thriving with other kids and safe yards in which to play. Downtown Boston was a ten-minute drive or a short subway ride away. During the summer, all the kids would spend the day at a local beach. If it wasn't a beach day, we'd play on the street kick the can, dodge ball, hide-and-seek or baseball. We were all called in for dinner at the same time, and we all came back out after dinner. Curfew was when the streetlights came on. As a kid back then, you didn't travel far; if you did, it was on your bike. Your bike took you everywhere. Parents didn't have two cars, and moms certainly wouldn't drive you anywhere unless it was a special occasion. Bike or walk, those were your choices.

When I was older, my friends and I would take the Blue Line into Boston to shop. We would go the Filene's, a department store; or Wild Pair, a funky shoe store for great shoes. Even today I can remember a particular pair. They were platforms with a rope heel, and about five inches of heel at that! Being only five-foot-two, I loved them, and saving my little paycheck from working at a clothing store was worth it. It was so much fun, and it felt so independent being in the big city!

My mom stayed home, and dad worked. I was the fourth child out of five. Frankie, Tommy, and Anne were older than I, and Paula came five years after me. Growing up, I have to say my mom made it look so easy. She cooked and cleaned, and generally took care of the house and the kids, pretty much on her own.

My dad, Frank, owned his own company, Eastern Flooring, in the next town over, in East Boston. It meant Dad working six to seven days a week. He would arrive home for dinner but didn't really help out much with us. It was a time when fathers provided money and support, but they weren't expected to really participate much in their children's lives.

I remember one night my mom had to go out to a PTA meeting. She cooked dinner beforehand, of course, and had us all bathed and ready for bed. All my dad had to do was walk us upstairs and put us to bed. Well, when mom came home later that night, my dad was asleep on the floor and all the kids were watching television. My dad had suggested that we all play the "nap game." That was my father's idea of watching the kids—playing the nap game, which he always won!

Living in a house with four teenagers was not always easy. My mom often tells me today, "Jodi, raising teenagers is like nailing Jell-O to the wall." I now know exactly what she means. To me, though, being a teenager was fun! Paula, who seemed so much younger than when I was a teen, seemed to relate more to mom than to Anne or I. Anne was two years older than I, with a small build, long and full blond hair (think Farah Fawcett), and lovely blue eyes. She and I got along pretty well, except when it came to borrowing clothes. That was like World War II. If she caught me wearing anything of hers without asking, she would get so mad. Clothes caused many battles in our house. However, we did not share the same friends or boyfriends, so the battles stopped with the clothing.

In addition to the clothes battles, Anne was messy and I was neat, and that caused problems since we three girls shared a room. Three girls in one room seems difficult but gave us ample opportunities for late-night conversations. We would talk about friends, boyfriends, and things we hoped mom would never find out about. The living arrangement developed a definite sense that we three would always be there for one another, an unspoken agreement that was realized later.

With five years between us, my younger sister, Paula, wasn't as involved with my daily life as I got older. She turned out to be taller than me, about five-foot-five, and had a muscular, solid build. We teased her that she looked a lot like Jennifer Lopez, except without the butt.

My two brothers, Frankie and Tommy, were always there for me. Frankie was eight years older; Tommy was four years older, so our parties and friends never really did cross paths. I sensed their care from a distance.

Frankie was the resident babysitter, I think mostly because he did not play sports and was around more than my brother Tommy, who was always playing hockey. My parents only went out on Saturday nights, and Frankie was the sitter... well, Frankie and his friends. They would sit around and listen to Carole King and Three Dog Night and Carly Simon and The Beatles, and let us do our thing.

Frankie had thick, curly, brown hair, and he's often let my sisters and I play with his hair and even put curlers in it. He had a great smile and was so easygoing and patient. I guess it was his way of controlling three young girls. With his medium build and brown eyes, he looked a bit unassuming but he was our big brother, and he was the one we all went to with our cares and concerns.

I remember one Christmas Eve in particular. I was young, still believing in Santa Claus, Frankie had come home from being out that evening with friends and noticed I was still awake.

"Can't you sleep, Jodi?" he asked.

"No, because Santa Claus is coming!"

"What are you thinking of especially?" he asked.

"I want a new Barbie doll and clothes for my doll." I showed him my cut-out pictures, lovingly scissored from the Sear "Christmas Wish Book" that had come in the mail weeks before. "And new bell bottoms!"

"I'm sure you'll get a lot of things on your list," Frankie assured me. We talked and talked and laughed about funny family memories and I eventually fell asleep, my big, strong brother watching over me.

His advice was always logical, and he had an amazing way of putting everything in perspective. You always left him feeling better. Being the oldest, he was the first to get a car, the first to get into a car accident, and the first to get caught drinking. He paved the way for the rest of us. As I look back, he was not a bad teenager at all.

I think the three girls were the real test for my parents. Or maybe just Anne and me! We managed to get into trouble on a weekly basis. I played intermural basketball after school, and worked at a nursing home in the kitchen. It seemed like I had a lot of extra time on my hands, though, and that is when I would get into trouble. My friends and I would steal beers from her dad's fridge and go down to the beach and drink. We always got caught. That, however, did not stop us. I enjoyed just hanging out with my friends, in the neighborhood or at the beach, listening to music and talking about boys.

Tommy was a hockey player and had the build to prove it. He was six feet, with straight brown hair, and a handsome face. His amazing dimples stood out when he smiled. It seemed he was always at the rink, and my mother was always driving him and his friends to a game or practice. My sisters and I also got dragged to the hockey rinks, forced to endure the cold bleachers and early morning hours. We didn't mind it if one of my brother's cute friends was playing.

He didn't give my parents much trouble at all. As a teenager, he was pretty focused, and hockey was his thing. He knew if he got into trouble, my parents would take his passion away. Tommy was the quietest of all five of us. When he did have something to say though, it was worth listening to, and he chose his words carefully.

Today my family is still close. Each summer we celebrate "Cava Fest" somewhere in the New England area; New Hampshire, Vermont, Maine, or Cape Cod. Each sibling takes a turn organizing the get-together, and all our families attend. We kids pair up and each take a night to prepare a meal, complete with themes, costumes, accessories, specialty drinks and games. And at the end of the weekend, there's a vote on the "best meal." One year we had a Tex Mex theme, with margarits, ribs, and piñatas all around. We did spaghetti and meatballs one year for our Italian theme. The winner has bragging rights for the next year. We are all taking different paths but value the camaraderie and respect we have for one another.

Besides family love, I met my "Prince Charming" early on. It was June 10, 1977, and I was fourteen years old. I knew Mark because he played hockey with my brother Tommy. I also was friends with his sister, Pam. It wasn't until Pam and her brothers had a party that we actually talked and got to know each other. Mark was sixteen, and I was immediately attracted to him and his beautiful blue eyes. I was nervous because he was older and very handsome. As the night progressed and we continued to get to know each other, we both realized a mutual attraction. I sat on his lap and our first kiss was like a fairy tale—magical.

With this background in mind, it was no surprise I was married at twenty-four to my prince and wanted to get pregnant right away. Like many dreams, this one took longer than I had planned.

Early on in our marriage, Mark and I lived in a second-floor apartment; there were many stairs to climb to get to our apartment. When I found out I was pregnant for the first time, I placed fresh carnations blue and pink alternating on each step. That was how I told him I was pregnant.

I was so happy and just couldn't wait to tell everyone. I did wait until twelve weeks, and everything seemed fine, so I told my family and friends.

But three weeks later, I felt a slight twinge and pain in my lower stomach. I brushed it off as nothing and continued in to work. As the day progressed, the pain stayed; it never got worse, but it never subsided either. I didn't tell anyone, but I was scared that something was wrong.

When I finally got home and told Mark, I started to cry hysterically. Deep down, I think I knew what was going on but just didn't want to admit it.

"Do you want to wait and see how you feel in the morning?" Mark asked me.

Reluctant yet worried, I nodded. "Yes, if I don't feel better then we'll go into the doctor's." The next day I started to bleed. I sat in the bathroom, holding my face in my hands, crying and shaking.

My worst fear was coming true.

I had a miscarriage. I was devastated—no explanation, no why, no reason. It just was. The doctors said, "It wasn't meant to be." Boy, did I hate hearing that!

Wasn't meant to be? is what I wanted to scream at them.

"Try again," was the reply. They seemed to have no clue how devastating a miscarriage was and how much it impacted a couple. For me especially, with my lifelong dreams from childhood about raising a family, it hit me really hard.

Of course we would try again. They tested Mark and I to see if we had anything genetic that would cause a miscarriage, but everything tested fine.

After the miscarriage, I felt inadequate, as if my womanhood was somehow less than other women's. One "friend" stood next to me at party and said, "Look at it this way. At least you can drink alcohol!"

The statement felt rude and uncaring.

With so many of our friends having children, I just wanted to be part of that world. I remember seeing pregnant women everywhere. At the grocery store, at the mall, in restaurants, at the movies. They all looked so beautiful, happy, and radiant!

I remember asking myself, *Why is it so difficult for me? Why are they pregnant and not me? Why is something so natural, so difficult?* Asking myself questions, doubting my body, my faith, and myself. I realized that I would never be able to get any answers, and therefore lived with the unknown. *Just let it go and trust God,* I kept telling myself. So we did, and we tried again.

In February 1989, we were living in East Boston, still in our small newlywed apartment. This time, no carnations. I simply told Mark, and we waited fourteen weeks before I told others. Two weeks later, I had my second miscarriage. No reason, no answer, no baby. This time I thought to myself, *My dream was not supposed to be this difficult.*

I can remember praying, asking God for help and guidance and His plan for my life. I felt I trusted Him and let it go, and He failed me; I was madder, sadder, and more confused. I knew I would be a mom someday, I visualized myself pregnant and carrying my children, but these days, the image was hard to hold on to.

The doctors performed more tests, and this time told me to wait a few months. Six months later, in August, I was pregnant. I thought, *How long before I tell anyone?* I had two ultrasounds, heard and saw the heartbeat, so I figured I was home free. Around fourteen weeks later, I again shared my news with friends and family.

I learned through two miscarriages just how difficult and trying life as an adult can be. I had to dig deep and find me, my faith, my strength, and my courage. I had friends, family, and Mark to comfort me, but this was the first time in my life that I had felt so sad and lonely, that I needed to help "me" get "me" okay again.

I thought I knew how hard life could be, but really had no idea at how deep I would have to dig and how far I would be tested.

> *Entrust your works to the Lord, and your plans will succeed.*
>
> —*Proverbs 16.3.*

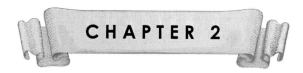

CHAPTER 2

The Plan

On May 8, 1990, my first child, Jordan Ashley Sampson, was born, and my long-held dream of family life finally began.

Jordan was delivered by C-section. We tried vaginal birth, but she was facing the wrong way. Babies are supposed to be delivered face-down, head first. Jordan was face-up. Dr. Testa, my obstetrician, would come in and turn her so she was face-down. I would push, and she would turn herself around again, face-up. That should have been my first indication: Jordan was not going to be an easy child!

And she wasn't. She ate well, slept well, but the minute she could talk and walk, I was in trouble. She was everywhere and into everything. Once she had a full vocabulary, there was no stopping her. I think I actually washed her mouth out with soap once. She said the F-word, so I put liquid soap on a facecloth and put it in her mouth. She never said that word again.

Every babysitter we had, she tortured. She would call them names, act up and cry every day I dropped her at daycare before heading to my job as a pattern-maker for Susan Bristol, a clothing company. I would peel Jordan off me and run out the door. She didn't like me working. At daycare, she would push other kids, and take leaves and throw them on others' heads.

Jordan had to be made aware of everything that was planned for the day, from breakfast to lunch to dinner to activities. If I wasn't the one to pick her up from school, I had to let Jordan know. One day I was running late from work, and my neighbor got Jordan for me. Of course, Jordan didn't know the plan. When I got home, she was so mad, yelling and screaming.

When she was six, we took her to a "talk doctor" (a counselor), looking for strategies to work better with Jordan's temper. We made sticker charts, mad pillows she could punch when she was upset, key words I was to use to help Jordan when she began to be mean to other kids. We employed hand gestures, daily charts, positive reinforcement involving small tokens. It was a lot of work! Somehow I couldn't help but think that spanking a child wasn't so wrong.

We all learned, grew, and worked our way through it. I knew Jordan's feistiness would be a benefit to her as an adult, if she learned to channel it properly. However, her feistiness was not a good quality for a six-year-old. But Jordan grew to be a very mature, organized, and focused teenager. She was still a bit difficult, but in a manageable way. I enjoyed her as a teen. She would share everything with me, even things I didn't particularly wish to hear.

Jordan knew I wasn't a "parent talker" and would not share with other parents what she told me. I was the "vault." I also did not react or overreact to the situations she told me about. I would use them as tools to see where she was and what she was thinking. I would say, "Well Jordan, what do you think about what he said?" or, "How would you have reacted differently?"

Not long after Jordan was born, I knew I wanted more children. It seemed I had the perfect life. I worked a few days a week, and my husband, Mark, had a great job as an outside salesperson for a software company. He sold to hospitals in the Midwest, and traveled every other week, three nights at a time, but was always home on the weekends. "The plan" I dreamed of was in place and working. We were saving for a house, and we lived in a nine hundred-square-foot apartment in the meantime. It was challenging, keeping it all together.

My next child, Kaitlin, was my Christmas gift! She was born on December 17, 1992. Again we attempted a vaginal birth. I pushed and her head would crown, then back in she would go. We did this for several hours before deciding a C-section would be better for Kaitlin as her heartbeat was becoming erratic. We used the same surgical site, and out came Kaitlin, silent and a lovely shade of purple. I couldn't see anything because a curtain covered me, but I heard Mark gasp. Moments later, we heard a cry: Kaitlin had had the umbilical cord wrapped around her neck. Again an indication of what this child would be like: resilient and tough as nails.

Kaitlin was my easy child. Nothing bothered her. At two years, nine months, she went off to preschool. I barely had the car in park and Kaitlin was unbuckled, out the door and up the stairs to school. She never looked back. Little Miss Independent, her favorite song was "She's a Wild One" by Shania Twain.

By 1994 with Mark traveling, me working, and the girls going every which way, we hired our first live-in nanny from Sweden. It helped calm things down, and I no longer had to rush to or from work to get to the babysitter. I had some help with all the housework and childcare.

But I guess I just wasn't busy enough, and thought a son would be the final part of the complete plan. I had two girls and really wanted a boy. Mark and I had talked about children, but he was a bit on the fence, still trying to figure out how he felt about it.

My periods had never been regular so for me, being late was semi-normal. In September 1995, I began to think there could be a reason, a very happy reason. I bought an EPT at the local Walgreens, and drove home, not sure myself if I wanted it to be positive or negative.

It was positive.

When Mark got home from work, he didn't even get a chance to get in the door and take off his coat. I hugged him and whispered in his ear, "We're pregnant!"

"How did that happen?" Men say the weirdest things. We both laughed and were happy.

Once I told Mark, I was relieved, and looking forward to being pregnant again. Even though we hadn't made a clear decision about having another child, we talked and decided it was a blessing, and something we agreed we wanted for each other and the family.

Two kids, pregnant, working four days, Mark traveling, and a live-in nanny from Sweden. All this happening in a nine-hundred-square-foot apartment. We were looking for a house as we saved our money; however, every time we went out and looked at houses, they all seemed way above our budget, and we felt we needed to save more money.

We really were not in any rush to leave our apartment. Mark's parents owned the two-family house, and generously rented one apartment to us for two hundred dollars a month. The lack of space was the only thing pushing us to get a house at this point. Still, the plan was unfolding, but it was becoming harder than I thought it would be.

Growing up, I remember my mom making it look so easy: five kids, her husband a small business owner who was never home and a balanced dinner on the table each night. Still, she always looked so happy. She knew her role in this world and in our family and took great pride in all she did for her family and her husband.

I now realize that she didn't have as many distractions as we have today. Our family lived a very simple life; never had new cars, never went on vacations, rarely went out to dinner as a family, unless someone graduated from school or got confirmed. Wealth, status, and material things where not very important to my mom, or my dad. Yet, they seemed happy.

I think it's harder today on parents because we compete with the outside world. We are constantly being pushed to attain wealth and a certain status. Even my children are told they need to play on "elite" teams, if they want to play sports in college. Elite teams means playing a sport all year round, traveling, which all means a large cost for families, and an enormous disruption in the family routine. The feeling that you have to "attain" or "participate" to get ahead in life were not themes threaded through my family life growing up.

I never realized all the hidden and unknowns my mom did for her family day in and day out would impact me as a parent and a wife. I often think about certain situations and think, *What would Mom do? What would she say?* When I do that, I always end up with the right answer and on top!

My parents had rules and you obeyed them. Not much was up for discussion, and "it's not fair" was one phrase my mom would not put up with. We where taught at a young age "life is just not fair, get used to it" in a kind, caring way.

As a adult, mother and wife, I never knew the "hidden" job my mom had of not only managing the house, but managing all the personalities and keeping peace in the house.

When we were all in school, my mom did work three days a week as a nurse's aide. She would walk home from work at 3:00 p.m., take a short nap, and be up to prepare dinner for all of us. She never, ever complained. I struggle to find that quality in me, and I only had three children and help with them.

My older brother Frankie was married by this time too, and we often turned to him and Chrissy for advice. Their children were a little older than ours, and they had gone through some of the things I was dealing with as a parent. They lived about five miles away from us, and we talked two to three times a week. To me, they both had logical and sound advice that, more importantly, made sense to me and I could implement.

Bedtime routine was one of them. I remember Frankie telling me, "Make sure you have a routine with your children. Bath, read a story, quiet rocking, holding time, and then bed. Whatever works for you and your children, just establish it and stick to it. Children thrive on routines and schedules." I understood this, as I thrived on schedules and routines as well.

Despite knowing the challenges ahead, Mark and I moved through this pregnancy with hope and excitement.

> *For who is God except the Lord? Who is a rock save our Lord? The God who girded me with strength and kept my way unerring*

> —*2 Samuel 22:32-33*

CHAPTER 3

The Devastation

ONE FRIDAY NIGHT IN MID-NOVEMBER, I was in our narrow, dark galley kitchen, preparing dinner, cooking Rice-a-Roni. On the dining room table was a wedding dress I'd made for my sister, Paula, who was getting married the following weekend. It was beautiful—sparkly, lacy, full of the promise of new life and new hope. I was feeling content.

The white wall phone, with its long, curly cord rang.

It was my sister Anne, the nurse. "Frankie has been taken to the hospital and his vital signs are not good."

"What does that mean?"

"Jodi, it's not good, just get to the hospital."

I remember trying to understand what my sister was saying and at the same time, looking for a "hopeful answer," but she couldn't give me one. She kept on spewing numbers at me, that mean nothing to me, but by the tone of her voice, it meant "bad news" to her. With her experience, Anne understood clearly what it meant to have "bad vital signs," but I had no clue.

My heart raced, my knees buckled and I was struck speechless. Mark was home and took the phone from me. I couldn't believe what I had heard. I just sat on the kitchen floor, crying and shaking. Mark finished the phone call and sat the floor next to me and held me tightly, crying. Mark knew exactly how I felt—his brother, Michael, had died thirteen years earlier at the young age of twenty-one on September 11, 1982.

Mark called his parents, and they came over to watch Kaitlin and Jordan. We drove to the hospital, not speaking. I was too frozen and frightened. What would we find at the hospital?

Hospitals scared me all my life. I can remember visiting my mom, I was about sixteen, in the hospital. She had a fibroid cyst removed, nothing real serious. I walked down the hall staring at the floor, so afraid to pick my head up and see something I did not want to see—blood or anything gruesome. I hated the smell of it. I hated the look of it. I just do not like blood, needles, IV poles, machines. All of them are very scary apparatuses to me.

When we got to the hospital, it was too late. Frankie was gone. *Where do I go from here? What do I do now?* I fell into that state of shock so common to survivors.

Two days later, we were present for the wake, two entire days at a funeral home in Winthrop. My whole family was in the greeting line: my parents, my siblings, his wife Chrissy, and their two children. The line of people waiting to get in was miles long and wound through the streets of the town. We saw Frankie's high school friends, old college friends, and dozens of others who knew my brother. We didn't leave the funeral home either night until 10 p.m.

Whoever thought this tradition was a good idea? I told Mark, "When I die, sit Shiva (we are not Jewish). Hang at our house, be comfortable, have people bring pastries from the north end of Boston, yes, cannoli! Drink, and talk about me! This business of standing, all dressed up, greeting, hugging, and kissing people is ridiculous, especially when you are not even in your own home!"

I no more wanted to talk to these people than I wanted to kiss and hug them. Many I did not know, nor did I care to know. Don't get me wrong, many people said just wonderful, heartfelt things about my brother that I wouldn't have heard, unless we had a wake. I was tired, mad, sad. I just wanted to be home, wrapped in a blanket with my own thoughts, blank and bleak as they may be.

My body was stiff and tight, but I wouldn't take any pain killers. Apparently, though, someone in the family was handing out Valium like an ice cream truck driver. But being pregnant and only three months along, I didn't want to jeopardize anything. I didn't dare take Motrin, Tylenol, or even a glass of wine or beer. I felt like the Tin Man in the Wizard of Oz, tight, stiff, and hollow inside.

We buried Frankie on his wife Chrissy's thirty-fifth birthday. Once the funeral was over, my body loosened up, no longer stiff but now shivering, unable to get warm. No matter what I had on, no matter how many blankets I put on the bed, I shook. Mark called my obstetrician, Dr. Testa, who warned him that my body had been dealing with the stress of everything and was just now letting go. Because of my history, it was likely I would miscarry, and that we should be prepared.

Two days later was Thanksgiving. I couldn't eat a thing, and I couldn't think of a thing to be thankful for. I prayed every morning, every day for answers. Why? Why did this have to happen to a great guy? Why did this happen to Chrissy? Thirty-five years old with two young boys, Frankie Jr., ten, and Nickie, six? What did we do wrong as a family to deserve such a tragedy?

The hardest part of losing someone we love was going on—going back to work and all of life's duties when all I felt like doing was crawling into bed. I hated feeling so sad, and it took such energy to do the simplest of tasks. As I did laundry, I found myself talking to God, looking for answers that would somehow make me feel better. As I cooked dinner, I would find myself praying to God for peace, comfort, and faith to go on. I found myself picking up the phone to call Frankie, only to dial the first three numbers and realize that he wasn't going to answer. I would see a truck that looked like his and follow it, thinking it could be him. What was wrong with me? I knew he was dead. Why was my mind so far behind reality? Was I losing my mind?

My uncertainty turned to unease at my first obstetrician appointment after Frankie's death. I felt worried about what the doctors would find. As I was driving to my appointment, my mind wandered once again to Frankie, I missed him so much it hurt my heart to breathe. I started to cry and just let it out for the thirty-minute car ride to the doctor's office. I managed to compose myself for my visit.

But once inside the office, when the nurse called my name, my heart began to race. I was so anxious—anxious about the baby and about my brother's death, a lot of mixed emotions going on all at the same time. We moved into an exam room. The nurse took my blood pressure and heart rate, then just stopped and looked at me.

"What is going on?" she asked. "Your blood pressure is very high, and your heart rate is over eighty."

I sat there and cried. I told her the whole story, and Dr. Testa, who had known all along, joined us in the room to offer his condolences and support. Once I calmed down, we were able to do an ultrasound, and I saw and heard the heartbeat! Despite all I had gone through, the baby's heartbeat was healthy and strong, and the ultrasound showed everything was progressing normally. What a relief!

Dr. Testa said, "You're extremely lucky not to have miscarried under the circumstances." I knew right then that this child would be a fighter and that God's hand was on this child's life and He would bless him or her. I left his office feeling better than I had in days.

It felt good to finally tell my family about my pregnancy now that I had reassurance from Dr. Testa that everything looked good. I was fifteen weeks along. They were elated. I believe it may have eased the pain of Frankie's death just a bit. When I told my mom, Pauline, she hugged me hard and whispered in my ear, "Jodi, this is the circle of life."

Little did I know how much this child would save me, my family and extended family, and cherished friends. I didn't yet know how much I needed this child. What a great sign of God's love for me and my family.

I never did wish to know the gender of the baby. I just felt inside that it was going to be a boy. I had lost two men who I loved dearly—Frankie and Mark's brother, Michael—and God is good. I believed He would give me another great guy to help me be great. So another C-section was planned for May 31, 1996, on my mom's birthday.

Michael Francis was born on May 31, 1996, at 10:00 a.m., with perfect Apgar scores and not a mark on his face, crying and beautiful. (An Apgar score refers to appearance, pulse, grimace, activity, and respiratory functions. It's more of a factor in vaginal births when a baby is squeezed through the birth canal.)

Michael was the first baby I tried to breastfeed. Previously, I had been very nervous with Jordan, plus, breastfeeding wasn't "in" in the 1990s. With Kaitlin, I thought I would be just too busy. How could I breastfeed and take care of a two-and-a-half -year old? So when Michael came along I thought, *This is my last chance.* I didn't want to have any regrets.

That day, once I was all sewn up and able to sit, Michael was handed to me swaddled in his blue blanket. His face looked beautiful to me. The nurse, who happened to be the same nurse in Dr. Testa's office during my first visit after my brother had died, was my nurse in the hospital. As she handed Michael to me, we both cried at how happy I was to have been blessed with a boy! That office visit had been so stressful, and now all the worrying and anxiety was over. I started breastfeeding right away and Michael latched on perfectly, starting a successful journey for both of us.

Life and my body were beginning to get back to normal, whatever that is with three kids, work, and daycare, cooking and cleaning—overwhelming. Mark had always said he liked to play man-to-man defense, and now that we were outnumbered, we needed to play zone. I realized the minute my feet hit the floor at 6:00 a.m. that nothing would be calm again until 10:00 or 11:00 at night. But as busy and as hectic as our lives were, I had a great feeling of inner peace.

At night, when I would lie in bed or in the rocking chair breastfeeding Michael, I often had weird thoughts pass through my mind. Thoughts of someone or something taking

Michael away from me. *I wasn't sure what these thoughts meant. Would someone kidnap him? From where? I left him in the baby room at childcare in the gym. Would someone take him from there? Would I lose him at the mall?* Unsettling as these thoughts were, I wasn't scared. I had an unexplainable peace and comfort that allowed me to remain calm, and the thoughts somehow didn't distract me. It would be two years before I understood where these thoughts came from.

In July 1997, we moved into a new house in a big new development. It felt wonderful to me, my dream of the big, happy family life coming true.

On a cool September morning later that year, we packed the kids into the mini-van.

"Where?" Michael burbled. He was one year, four months old, toddling stage, just learning to really run.

"It's a surprise!" I answered. His brown eyes opened wide; Michael loved surprises.

We were headed to the annual Meditech Picnic. Mark's company transformed his company's plush greens into an amusement park. They had trolley cars, flying swings, go-karts, tethered air balloons, face painting, sand art, treasure hunts, sack races, and sand castle making with piles of sand to dig in. Food was everywhere—lobsters, burgers, hot dogs, ice cream, cotton candy.

Michael squealed with delight.

He ran from one ride to another. The flying swings where his favorite.

"I want to go!" he said.

"I have to go with you," I explained. "You're too young to go by yourself. Let me hold you on my lap."

"I wanna go, like Jordan and Kaitlin!" He was so mad, he wanted to go on by himself. I finally managed to convince him; he could hurt himself, and he reluctantly went on with me.

Our feet hung free, swinging in the air, and we flew around and around. Michael loved it. At the end of the day, we buckled him into his car seat with cotton candy in one hand and a candy apple in the other. We barely made it out of the parking lot and he was fast asleep. It was such a great sight, a tired and satisfied baby.

That Halloween was our first holiday there as a family. Our family had always loved Halloween and loved getting dressed up. I especially loved it because I made all the costumes for the kids—and myself!

That year I was Cruella Deville, complete with Dalmatians sewn into pockets, sitting on my shoulders and on my back. We dressed Michael as a lion with a hood that velcroed under his chubby cheeks and yarn for a full mane. A brown nose and whiskers completed his look. Jordan was dressed as a leopard, and Kaitlin was dressed as a princess.

Mark and I took turns taking the children out trick-or-treating, and that year Mark stayed home to hand out candy and I went through the neighborhood with the kids. At a year and a half old, Michael was in a baby carriage, and the girls ran alongside.

When we got to the first house's walkway, Michael practically jumped out of the carriage and ran up to the front door. Michael loved to get candy and had the biggest smile ever. He wouldn't even make it back to the carriage before the candy was unwrapped and in his mouth and all over his face. I remember how fast he got out of breath running up and down the long walkways.

Our old neighborhood was more urban, where the houses were so close you could open up the window and touch the next house. There were three apartments per house, so one house would get you a lot of candy. In the new suburban neighborhood, there was a lot of running and distance between houses and candy! However, that didn't deter Michael; he was up for the challenge and he ran and ate his way through the neighborhood. At the end of the night, Michael sat on the living room floor with his bag of candy all around him, stuffing his face. It was a great night!

Three kids, *check!* Brand new house in a great development with all new houses being built all around us, *check!* I had all the bathrooms and bedrooms I would need, a great backyard, and a two-car garage, *check!* I was living my dream again. "The plan" was back on. But my marriage was falling apart.

One Thursday night in November of 1997, when Mark got home from his travel, we had a major tiff.

"I've been taking care of the house and the kids all week," I said. "Please, let's go out to dinner."

"No, I'm too tired, and I've been on the road all week. I just want to stay home," Mark said.

"I need a break!"

Mark glared at me. "Jodi, I've eaten out at restaurants every night this week. I want to stay home! Really."

"You have no idea how hard I work here while you're gone. The kids are just overwhelming," I said. I tried to explain myself, but it wasn't going well.

"And you have no idea how stressful it is for me out there. The damn airports, the delayed flights, the pressure from clients." Mark jerked his tie off. "And the second I walk in the door, the kids are all over me! There's no break at all."

"Well, they're your children too," I countered. And we were off on another argument.

I felt Mark was being insensitive to my need for a break, and he felt I was wrongheaded about insisting on going out when he just got home. In the midst of everything, Mark and I had let "us" slip away. We had devoted ourselves to careers, attaining the great house, kids, grief, anger, and pain, but had left nothing for each other. We disagreed and argued about everything—children, food, and finances, even what we wore.

In January of 1998, Mark and I decided it was best if he moved out. We weren't sure where this move would lead us, but it was all I could think to do.

Once Mark moved out, we were both able to focus on the real problems and think clearly. We went to counseling and talked, and talked and talked. Through all our sessions and time alone with each other, we found that we both wanted the same thing—we just needed help getting there. We needed time to be together, being flexible with each other's plans, communicating with each other, respecting each other's differences, and being willing to give up some part of ourselves for the other.

The final outcome for Mark and I was that we loved each other and neither of us wanted a divorce. We just needed to slow down and put "us" on the list of things to do. It took a lot of patience and give and take to mend "us," but I feel we both learned so much about each other. We grew from the experience. Mark and I renewed our wedding vows and began our journey once again. Mark moved back home in March of that year.

> *So faith, hope and love remain, these three: but the greatest of these is love.*
>
> *—1 Corinthians 13:13*

CHAPTER 4

There Goes a Tractor

IN FEBRUARY OF '98, KAITLIN came down with some sort of virus and vomited constantly. She considerately passed it on to me, then Jordan, and finally to Michael. Everyone seemed to recover fully but Michael. For a month, it was doctor appointments, emergency room visits, specialists, and gastroenterologists, all trying to figure out what was wrong with Michael. He vomited constantly and was lethargic. He lost weight. Some days he would seem to be better, and then the next day be very sick again. Every night I prayed, "God give me answers. Put the right people in my life so that I might figure this out."

In March, I'd even made a journal entry about Michael being sick; it had gone on for so long. Finally, in April, I made an appointment with a pediatric gastroenterologist to help figure out what was wrong with Michael. I put Jordan on the school bus, and my friend Jean came by to take Kaitlin to preschool. Mark was away on business, and I kept him informed of what was going on with Michael by phone.

As I drove to Salem that Wednesday morning, I was both scared and relieved. I knew in my heart that I was being pointed in the right direction; unfortunately, I had an uneasy feeling that the direction was not a good one. After a full exam, the doctors could not find the source of Michael's illness and suggested we go to Massachusetts General Hospital for a comprehensive battery of tests: CBC (complete blood count), electrolytes, chest X-rays, upper GI, barium swallow, bone scan, and brain scan.

The gastro doctor told me, "We're very concerned because Michael has lost thirteen percent of his body weight, and he's now malnourished. We can't find the source, and this is worrisome." His look was grave; I knew then that this was a serious problem.

Michael lay in my arms as we talked. He was listless, inactive, and quiet. My heart tightened, and I felt sick to my stomach. The exam room tried to be cheerful with its yellow walls, but outside, the day was typical Massachusetts February—cold, gray, and dreary. It mirrored what I was feeling just then.

"We'll need to do all of these tests to get to the bottom of Michael's illness. MGH will be able to figure this out, don't worry. You'll be home by the weekend."

Finally I was getting somewhere! As we were finishing up with our visit, I told the doctor, "I want a head scan done."

"Why?"

"I think Michael may have a brain tumor."

"I'll order the scan, but Michael doesn't present as a child with a brain tumor."

At Massachusetts General Hospital, we were placed in the pediatric ER, away from adults and regular patients. The doctors asked me the same questions over and over again.

Was Michael's birth normal? Were there any complications?

At what age did he start to eat regular food? Sit up? Walk, crawl, stand, sleep through the night?

Was he immunized? Any history of heart disease in your families?

Is anyone else in your family ill? How did Kaitlin and the rest of the family get sick? How long had Michael been sick? What was eating then? Is he allergic to milk? The questions just went on and on and on as the doctors tried to narrow down the symptoms and possible causes.

Michael and I just sat there and answered them. After a few hours, Michael felt better and ran up and down the floor. The test results were all coming back normal, with no clue as to what was ailing Michael.

"Since nothing is obvious from the tests, can we do a head scan?" I asked. The doctors agreed to schedule a scan. I called Mark, who was just about to get on a plane to head home to Boston, and told him what was going on. "Please come directly to MGH, and hurry!" I also called my sister Anne, who just happened to be working that day, to meet me in the emergency room.

I had no sooner hung up the phone when hospital transport was there to take us to the CT scan. As Michael was wheeled down the hall and into the CT scan, an emergency stretcher flew by us, pushing us aside. There had been a severe car accident, and many victims needed a CT scan asap. I was a little relieved. I wanted answers, but was so worried about what the answers would be. Michael was wheeled back to the pediatric emergency room, where we both sat, waiting.

As we sat waiting to be called again, the time seemed to go by very slowly. We'd arrived at MGH about noon, and finally, about 7 p.m., Mark and Anne made it in. I was so happy to see their faces. Soon, transport arrived again to take Michael, Mark, and me for the scan.

I went into the scanner with Michael, donning my lead-weighted apron for protection as Michael was strapped into the cold, white sterile shoot. His little head was gently placed in a small cylinder, and they taped his forehead to help him stay still. They wrapped his body with blankets because it was cold in there. The only things visible were his tiny hands. And they were so tiny! He was only twenty-two months old and had to go through this ordeal.

I stood beside the scanner as they positioned his head for the imaging. I was cold, tired, scared, relived, and nauseous all at the same time. I held his hands and prayed, not sure what I was praying for. "Jesus, help us." That's all I had.

⁂

Within ten minutes, we were all back in the exam room. I was on edge, noticing the heavy wooden door, the tiny window showing the night's darkness outside. A counter strewn with medical implements and medications hung on one side of the room. Mark, Anne, Michael, and I huddled on the chairs, the small TV in the room silent. It was cold, and both Michael and I had blankets draped over us. The overhead light was bright, too bright.

At about 11 p.m., a knock came at the door. Within seconds, staffers crowded into the room with us—the attending ER doctor, the on-call neurology doctor, Dr. Ebb, a pediatric oncologist, and the ER nurse. Wearing scrubs and stethoscopes, draped around their necks like snakes, looked so intimidating. The room shrank under their presence.

I felt cold, so cold.

One doctor finally spoke up. "We found a mass in Michael's head, in the right occipital lobe. We need to do further tests to determine how extensive it is, and most likely, he'll need surgery."

Great crowds followed Him and He cured them there.

—Matthew 19:2

CHAPTER 5

Why, God, Why?

"Is it cancer?" Mark asked.

"Many brain tumors in small children are, but we won't know for sure until we do further tests."

My brain told me that meant there's a chance it may not be cancer. But at the same time I wondered, *Why was Dr. Ebb, the pediatric oncologist here?*

"Most brain tumors are fast-moving and aggressive," Dr. Ebb told us. "He'll need surgery, and the unfortunate reality is most brain tumors are malignant. This will mean chemotherapy, radiation, and many surgeries."

I looked at all the doctors' faces and could see in their eyes that this was a grave situation. I didn't cry, I just sat there like a statue, no questions, no "how did this happen?"—

nothing. I could barely breathe. I wanted to leave that room, and more importantly, I wanted the doctors to leave that room. With Michael in my arms, my knees buckled, and I felt like I was going to hit the floor. I dropped into the chair, sobbing, clinging to Michael, so frail and small, wrapped in his blankets.

The doctors all left the room, having changed our future forever.

I felt as though someone had just kicked me in the stomach about a hundred times.

Hospital transport came to get Michael up to a room. I climbed on the stretcher and lay down next to him, unwilling to let him out of my sight or reach. Mark and Anne walked behind us.

I looked down at little Michael, so tired and almost asleep, too young to understand what was happening, too sick to realize what was happening.

Once settled in the room, the doctors and nurses came back again to talk some more, and review Michael's vital signs. All the doctors and nurses were taking more labs. Michael had an IV so they where constantly checking all his chemistry. But I do remember they were mostly observing Michael and Mark and me.

I now look back and see how concerned they were not just for Michael, but for Mark and I. Always asking if we needed anything, could they send in a priest, a social worker with vouchers for food, and just someone to talk to about anything. Volunteers brought in therapy dogs, nurses that practiced "energy healing" (Reiki), constantly checking in on us, most likely checking Michael and our demeanor.

That first night Mark and I slept in the other bed, together. They put us in a room for two patients, but because of the severity of Michael's illness, they did not put another patient in the bed, another clue, as I look back. Mark and I fell asleep very late, and I remember being woken up in the middle of the night maybe around four-ish. Transport was coming to take more pictures of Michael's head, another MRI. After the MRI and we were back upstairs, Mark and I stood in the middle of Michael's room, with its beautiful view of the Charles River and the moonlight sending silver rays on the water, and we held each other and cried together for a long time

It was the start of years of waiting and worrying at the hospital.

The next few days were filled with waiting and watching in Michael's hospital room. I noticed an odd calmness even with many people going in and out of the room. Buzzers went off, alarms sounded, and a sense of concern from all who entered, both staff and family, permeated. The staffers were there for mostly observation, checking in on us. Like the calm before the storm, a strange ominous aura filled the room.

Many of my family were there with us, and they all came with their own questions and concerns. My sister Paula brought up the topic of nutrition.

"I know you buy your vitamins and supplements from a friend, Elaine from Shaklee. What do you think she'd have to help Michael?"

"I don't know, but that's a good idea," I said.

"I'll talk to her," Paula said. "Maybe see what Shaklee has to offer Michael along the lines of vitamin supplements. And what about his water?"

Mark chimed in, "I agree. The water he drinks is important. What kind of regulations are there for bottled water?"

"I've read about juicing too," Paula said. "It's supposed to be really good for ridding your body of the toxins that accompany chemotherapy. I'll look into a machine for you to juice at home."

We all wanted to do something and when Paula mentioned nutrition, it was easy for me to wrap my hands around. Mark also started to look into different fruits and veggies to juice to help Michael; so it was a team effort, and Mark, Paula, and I felt like we could actually do something to help Michael.

We spent the next couple of days in the hospital, inundated with doctors, nurses, surgeons and, of course, family and friends. They were running more tests and needed everyone in place before performing the surgery on Michael's brain.

A doctor told us, "It's a bulky tumor, and it's already metastasized down into his spine. We have a lot of questions about how to perform the surgery because in a child, especially, the space to work with is so small. We need to consult neurology, and we need to determine how much surgery this small child can endure."

The doctors were pretty much leaving Michael alone, except to come in and out of the hospital room and observe him. There where residents, attending interns, nurses, and neurology fellows, all coming in to observe and look at Michael. This went on for days, as they strategized the best way to perform this surgery. It was a Wednesday when Michael was diagnosed; they didn't operate until the following Monday.

Dr. Ebb was the main doctor we spoke with. "The Black Cloud," that was what I called Dr. Ebb behind his back. He wasn't a bad-looking man by any means. He wore khaki-colored Dockers and a plaid shirt most every day, and his brown eyes hidden behind his wire-rimmed glasses. He was caring and compassionate, but I couldn't help but feel hatred for the man who had delivered so much bad news to us!

We had multiple meetings with all the doctors and hearing everything they had to say: *may not survive, blood clot, cannot stop the bleeding, the head is very vascular, tumor too difficult to remove.*

With each meeting, I grew weaker and more helpless. During one meeting, Dr. Ebb, the pediatric oncologist, was talking and talking, and I just could not take it any longer. I stood up and said, "Stop, stop talking, I cannot hear anymore!"

Dr. Ebb tried to show me a picture of a central line that would be surgically inserted into Michael's chest for administration of chemotherapy and nutrition. He handed me a piece of paper with a picture of what it would look like. Michael would have two pieces of tubing hanging out of the left side of his chest. One port would be for chemotherapy, and the other would be for TPN, a nutritional supplement that would sustain him during chemotherapy.

"The chemo will make him very ill," Dr. Ebb said. "He most likely will not be able to eat."

As I stared at the piece of paper, I got so enraged; I threw the paper at Dr. Ebb! I couldn't look at it anymore. I just kept repeating, "No, no, no, get away from me." It was too much for me to hear, understand, digest. Dr. Ebb calmly got up and left.

⁂

One day of that awful week, my cousin Carol came to visit me in the hospital. She brought me her Bible and picked out scriptures about healing for me to read. She circled them all in the Bible and told me to continue to read them, even though I had never read the Bible before this. It was a beautiful book—the burgundy cover matching the burgundy satin bookmark ribbon. I began to carry it with me, everywhere. I felt its comforting weight in my purse, in my hand, at my side nearly every minute of the day.

Nights before bed, I read from my Bible, its burgundy, hammered-leather cover growing worn beneath my fingers. The pages began to show wear, and many of them were marked with dates and names of people I was praying for (1/2000-Joe and Jean, 5/2001-Paula). I took comfort from the simple words, never suspecting that I would be needing its inspiration so desperately in the days to come.

It was my only hope.

The last meeting before the scheduled surgery was with three surgeons, Dr. Rob Freidlander, Dr. Paul Chapman, and Dr. Ed Smith. I felt physically and mentally beat up, and I just couldn't sit through another meeting. I had asked my sister Anne to go with Mark to the meeting. She was a nurse and could help Mark and I understand the medical lingo. So Anne and Mark met with the three surgeons while I stayed in the room with Michael.

I still remember the look on their faces as they returned—white and petrified.

"What did they say?" I asked.

"Nothing new," Mark said. "Just the same precautions that they told us before. Not much really."

There's something he's not telling me. But I didn't push.

Anne made very little eye contact. "I helped Mark understand what they were saying, but, uh, now I have to get back to work and check on one of my patients." Normally,

Anne talks and talks and talks—this was new for her. She abruptly left the room.

I knew they had heard terrible outcomes from the surgeons, and I was grateful for the moment, not to know, not to carry that awful knowledge in my heart yet. I wasn't ready for it.

"I want to head home and get more clothes," Mark said. As he left the room and walked down the hall, I forgot to ask him to bring me some clothes too. I ran after him and noticed that he did not take the elevators, but went into the stairwell. We were on the seventeenth floor. No way was he walking down seventeen flights of stairs.

I cautiously walked to the door of the stairwell and, on my tiptoes, peeked through the small glass window. The door was heavy gray steel and cold, ugly, and hard to open. The stairwell was painted gray as well, and there sat my Mark, bent over with his hands over his face. He was crying uncontrollably, rocking back and forth.

I had never seen my husband like this before, and I knew he felt as helpless and scared as I did. Whatever he had heard in that meeting devastated him, and I knew I didn't want to hear it. I just stood there, frozen, staring.

He's my rock. How can he fall apart? What am I supposed to do now? He has to be the strong one, he has to hold it together!

I had no ability to move my body or console him; I was just totally paralyzed. My stomach twisted, as if someone had a tight grip on my insides. As I watched, Mark finally got up and headed down the seventeen flights of stairs.

As my husband walked down into the grayness, I knew then and there that we were in a battle much bigger than I could realize.

> *Jesus said to them in reply, Have faith in God Amen,*
> *I say to you, whoever says to this mountain, be lifted up and thrown into the sea and does not doubt in his heart but believes that what he says will happen, it shall be done for him. Therefore I tell you, all that you ask for in prayer, believe that you will receive it and it shall be yours.*

> —*Mark 11:22–24*

CHAPTER 6

Hospital as Home

MONDAY MORNING CAME, AND MICHAEL was wheeled into the operating room. Total surgery time was estimated to be ten to twelve hours.

My parents, Pauline and Frank, were there, along with Mark's parents, Stan and Arylne. Anne came too, and our best friend, Joe. Jordan and Kaitlin were home with my friend Jean.

The group of us trudged across the street to Harvard Gardens for lunch to fill some of the wait time. I just pushed my food around on my plate. It seemed like someone had a vise and was squeezing it in my stomach. We ended up crowding into the waiting room on that seventeenth floor. There were so many of us; we all wanted to be together when the surgeons came to let us know of the outcome. I sat on the couch with Mark in silence, praying and hoping that the surgeons would come through the door with good news.

It seemed like forever passed before the surgeons came to deliver the news, but it was about eight hours; evening had come.

The surgeons were brief. "Michael has done well. We were able to remove the tumor, and bleeding was minimal. We took out as much as we could. However, it had spread to other portions of the brain, vital to its function. The cancer that has spread will need to be eradicated with chemotherapy."

I just stood there with my mouth open.

"This may sound like bad news, but it's actually pretty good. We're very happy we were able to remove the tumor, it was as big as a tennis ball."

Michael would be in the intensive care unit for a few days, then back on Ellison 17 for a few weeks.

All I wanted to do was see Michael with my own eyes, to make sure he was fine. Mark and I were finally admitted into the Pediatric Intensive Care Unit (PICU).

"Michael, Michael, how's my Michael," I said when we got to his bed.

Michael lay on his side with his tiny head all wrapped with gauze. There was a tube in his nose, many, many IVs coming out of both arms, a catheter, a central line placed in his chest, and EKG leads all over his body. But even with all the apparatus, his eyes were bright, and he smiled at us.

"Michael, wake up, we're here now. How are you?" I had a hard time finding a clear place to put my hands on him.

"My head hurts," he said. He talked! What a relief!

I wanted to crawl onto that gurney and hug him. He was talking, saying that his head hurt, and his hands and feet all worked well. He had some life in his eyes, life that I hadn't seen in the last few weeks. He looked perfectly normal, except for the big bandage wrapped around his head.

Mark and I took turns holding his hands. He was in and out, but talking some and making sense. We were able to stay for a few minutes, but then the nurse had us leave.

"In the PICU," she explained, "you have one-on-one nursing care around the clock. He'll never be alone, and when the shift changes, another nurse will be in charge. Don't you worry; he's in good hands."

"That makes me feel better. I think I can leave him and go upstairs to the floor, knowing that," I said. "Thank you, thank you so much!"

When Mark and I pushed that big silver exit pad to leave the PICU, I felt relieved. Maybe I could breathe a bit better, finding consolation in the unknown becoming known. My chest started to loosen, and my heart felt lighter, just for a moment.

> *And whatever you ask in My name, I will do, so that the Father may be glorified in the Son. If you ask anything of me in my name, I will do it.*
>
> *—John 14:13–14*

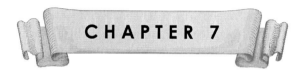

Standing Firm

A FEW DAYS LATER, MICHAEL was able to go back to "his room" in Ellison 17. Four days later, D.r Ebb sat us down and gave us the bottom line: Michael had a PNET (Primitive Neuroectodermal Tumor) which, in civilian-speak, meant a fast-growing mass. His words somehow made it through the buzz in my own head as he spoke to us quietly. "The mass has spread to inoperable parts of his brain, and cancer cells are floating in his spinal fluid. I'm sorry, but the prognosis is not good."

"What about the chemo? Radiation?" I asked. The "normal" treatments for cancer seemed a little logical.

Ebb shook his head. "Radiation isn't an option as he is so young. It would have irreversible effects on his growth and development. And chemotherapy has never been able to completely eradicate this type of cancer. Given this, it looks like Michael is only likely to survive six months."

Numb and silent, I just sat there and cried. I remembered when Michael was first born, and my thoughts of having someone take him away. I now know that God was preparing me for this news. Some*one* wasn't going to take Michael: some*thing* called *cancer* was going to try to take Michael from us.

In early May, after being in the hospital for nearly a month, we were finally allowed to go home. My world had been completely turned upside-down. I didn't know where to begin. I had stopped working as a patternmaker for Susan Bristol and knew all my time would be devoted to Michael. I was to expect visiting nurses, home health aides, and all types of medicine and medical supplies. I was overwhelmed and confused.

The first night a visiting nurse came to our home to help us set up Michael's pump. It would supply Michael with nutrients through one of the ports in his central line. The pump would be hooked up to Michael at 6:00 p.m. every night and run twelve hours, until 6:00 a.m. the next morning. It had to be flushed out with Heparin first, and then a saline solution, before we could administer the nutrients.

Within a few minutes of the nurse being at my home, my kitchen pantry had been transformed into a hospital supply closet, complete with syringes, tubing, pumps, sharps containers, alcohol wipes, saline, needles, and Heparin. Not only did I have to house this stuff, I had to do inventory! The home care company that supplied us would call once a week to and ask what supplies we would need for the upcoming week, so I would have to keep a careful inventory.

A visiting nurse would come twice a week to clean and examine Michael's central line. Since the line was inserted into a major artery leading directly to Michael's heart, it was crucial that it not get infected as an infection could kill him. Keeping that sight infection-free was top priority! This meant no water anywhere near the sight. No baths, just a shower. I would wrap his body with saran wrap to keep the sight protected, and shower around it. No pools, no beaches, no sand! We were very limited, and very cautious with Michael's care.

I hated hospitals and medical stuff, but it now had invaded our home. The visiting nurse was there to demonstrate how the pump worked as, for the most part, this would be our responsibility. Mark and I would have to hook up the TPN to Michael's central line.

I felt so uncomfortable being a medical caregiver for me son. I never felt uncomfortable as a mother for any of my children, but this was way over my head. I was nervous as the nurse said good-bye and walked out my front door.

You're kidding me! I can't do this!

My calm, comfortable home had turned into a scary place; I didn't feel comfortable being home alone with Michael, even though Mark was there. I put Michael in his crib that first night but could not leave him alone. It was large enough and I was tiny enough that I climbed into his crib with him and laid beside him, too scared and tired to move. Until now he'd had nurses and doctors watching over him 24/7. Now I had to be vigilant, to see and react to his condition, things that I knew nothing about. I just wanted to be next to him.

The poor baby finally fell asleep, and I got out of the crib. I went downstairs to join Mark, and poured myself a glass of wine. But I couldn't sit still, and I ran up and down the stairs to check on him Michael. As Mark and I headed to bed, we heard his pump alarm going off.

"What do we do?" I asked frantically. "I can't fix it!"

"Let's call the nurse," Mark said, and sure enough she politely answered the phone and said she'll be right over.

Within a few minutes, my doorbell rang and there she was. She simply replaced our faulty pump with a new one. Michael slept through all of it.

Exhausted, I fell into bed, grabbed my Bible off the nightstand and began to read. Carol had shown me thirty-eight healing scriptures that clearly described Jesus's healing power and bookmarked them to refer back to. I'm not entirely sure I understood what I was reading, but as I read, I felt calmer and more able to have peace in my heart. I read them out loud as Mark lay beside me.

> *Great crowds came to him, having with them the lame, the blind, the deformed, the mute and many others. They placed them at his feet and he cured them.*
>
> *—Matthew 15:30*

After a few verses, I looked over; Mark was asleep and I was on my way too. By the time I had finished reading all thirty-eight scriptures, I was already half asleep.

The next day began at 6:00 a.m. I unhooked Michael from his pump. Shortly after, everyone was up and the phone began ringing—doctors, hospitals, friends and family, all calling to help and check on Michael. Child services called to schedule an occupational therapist and a physical therapist to come to the house for Michael. And did I need an aide to come for a few hours a day? Since Michael had gone into the hospital, my mother came to my house almost daily to do laundry.

I sat down to figure out Michael's medicine and how to organize and remember what he needs and when he needs it. I realized I needed to make a chart of all the medicine Michael had to take, some every six hours, some one time daily, another twice, and yet another had a tapered dose. I couldn't keep it all straight; this was so difficult! I didn't understand all that was going on and how I would cope with all this new stuff. I used to work four days, take care of three kids, cook, clean and manage my home while Mark traveled. Now I couldn't even sit down and figure out a medicine chart!

There were so many people in my life who wanted to help me, who I *needed* help from, and I let them help. Allowing help was a new concept to me. I thought that the old saying of "It takes a village" is true!

One thing I'd come to realize is, I needed to "check out" occasionally. That meant I had to go upstairs to my bedroom, close and lock the door, and sit quietly. When things got to be too much for me and I felt overwhelmed, I checked out, went to my bedroom, sat on my bed and read my thirty-eight scriptures in an effort to find peace and tranquility, away from the hectic circumstances of the moment. As the weeks went by, my Bible became a bit frayed, the thin pages getting worn and marked-up with my underlining, some highlighting, and even some of Michael's scribbles. Water marks from tears and coffee stained. The Bible became a physical touchstone of comfort and serenity for me in a world where I was tested and tried more than I'd ever imagined.

> *And he said, What is impossible for human beings is possible for God.*
>
> —*Luke 18:37*

That morning, D.r Ebb's office called to explain Michael's chemotherapy schedule and when we would begin. *Boy,* I thought to myself, *they don't leave you alone, home one day and already chemo! Yuck!* We set up Michael's chemo schedule every week for six weeks. Michael would be in the hospital for two days each time to receive it.

I remember the first day of chemo. Michael was hooked up to an IV that would deliver it. As the nurse came in with the drugs, I had envisioned a container with skulls and crossbones. I thought about all the precautions we took as parents to protect our children from harmful substances and environments. Installing locks on kitchen cabinets that housed cleaning supplies that could be lethal if ingested, keeping all medicine high in a cabinet out of the reach of children, avoiding smokers, making sure we had no lead paint in our house, choosing appropriate toys with no small, removable parts—we had a house that was baby-proofed to the max!

Yet there I sat as I watched a nurse administer poison to my son. I just couldn't wrap my head around it! Of course, the difference was that this poison was saving Michael's life and hopefully not harming him in the meanwhile. Would the chemo cause Michael to light up like some glow-in-the-dark toy, or start violently vomiting? None of the two happened, but I learned just what the poison could do.

And the poisons were several: Vincristine, Cisplatin, Cyclophosphamide, Oral Etoposide. Vincristine side effects included loss of hair, jaw pain, muscle weakness, tingling in the hands, droopy eyelids, and a chance of sterility. Cisplatin could cause nausea, vomiting, and hearing loss. Cyclophosphamide included side effects of nausea, vomiting, hair loss, low blood counts, and bladder irritation. Oral Etoposide could cause nausea, vomiting, hair loss, and low blood counts.

Many of the side effects wouldn't show up right away, if at all. It was always a matter of "wait and see." Not that the side effects didn't matter, of course, but they were always secondary to the larger problem of the cancer.

Michael received all of these medications through the IV. Despite my worries and fears, that day was actually pretty uneventful. We returned home after the two-day stay, but Michael, as could be expected, just didn't feel well. He wanted to be held all the time, so Mark and I took turns holding him. He slept a bit, but otherwise just tossed and turned. It just seemed he could not get comfortable. He was nauseous, so Zofran was prescribed, which seemed to help. We continued the protocol for the six weeks, as scheduled.

⧈

Mark and I had started making changes right away in our diet, even before Michael came home from the hospital. I purchased a water filtration system because I didn't feel comfortable even with bottled water. We were already a "vitamin-taking family;" we just added things like Omega 3, EPA, DHA and ALA, and fish oil to Michael's supplements. We would squeeze the oil out of the capsules and add it to his juice. They had such great health benefits, especially in the fight against cancer.

Just as Paula promised, she did the research and we bought a juicer. We juiced anything form carrots, apples, celery, lemons, pears, kale, to oranges. Anything we could possibly get Michael to sip. We put an ounce in a medicine cup, and tried to have him sip it. We had read so much about a healthy diet and how it can help fight cancer, we were compelled to try it.

We tried to give him some carrot juice. I put some in a medicine cup, which was only one ounce, and tried to get

Michael to sip it. He sipped it and spit it out, so we tried adding apples or pears to sweeten it up—still nothing. I then gave some of our new concoction to Jordan and Kaitlin—and they spat it out!

They both said, "This is awful I can't believe you're making Michael drink this!" So we had to experiment with different veggies and fruits to find something palatable. We had a hit with carrots, oranges, and lemons. It wasn't a big hit, but at least he didn't spit it out. We continued juicing, eating only organic foods, and giving him vitamin supplements. Everything Michael had we tried too! He was never alone in our search for healthy, nutritious foods and vitamin supplements.

Needless to say, Michael was not interested in any of our remedies and often refused to drink them. He felt awful and I guess the thought of drinking anything, let alone juice with fish oil added to it, was not happening. It just shows you how desperate Mark and I were in helping cure Michael.

For those six weeks, I was at the hospital every week for two nights for Michael to receive his chemotherapy. There was a team of nurses who always took care of Michael, and they tried to always give us the same room. After being in the hospital for a month and then back every week, I got used to the hospital as my second home, eating in the same cafeteria, seeing the same people. The guy who parked my car, Mac, knew our names. The lady in the café knew my name; the volunteer Abby, an older woman, always found us, and brought Michael candy and toys. Odd as it sounds, the hospital became so familiar to me. Where all the vending machines were, where to find the best coffee and how late the Coffee Connection stayed open. I knew it all.

At the end of the six-week protocol, Michael was scheduled to receive another MRI to see if anything in his head had changed.

In mid-June, after six weeks of chemo, Dr. Ebb, "the Black Cloud," did the MRI. Our hospital room on Ellison 17 of Massachusetts General Hospital now seemed like our second home. Mark was traveling on business, so my in-laws, Stan and Arlyne, and one of Michael's team nurses, Elise, waited with me for the results. She worked on discharge papers as we all sat together, silent and nervous.

I sat in the world's most uncomfortable chair, holding Michael. He was lethargic and half-asleep. It was just starting to get dark, about 8 p.m. The darkness outside the hospital windows seemed to press in on me.

Dr. Ebb, his plaid shirt mostly blue today, entered the room with a very serious look in his eyes. My stomach dropped; I knew the news would not be good

He stood across from me and leaned up against the closet. "I'm sorry to say that the MRI showed no change in Michaels' cancer. Nothing is different from the first MRI. We'd hoped to see some indication that this protocol of chemo is working, but we're not seeing it."

"Well, maybe it just takes a longer time?" I asked.

Dr. Ebb shook his head. "The protocol is very specific. If you don't see any results after administering the chemo, then it most likely will not be effective and you should find an alternative."

I couldn't believe, what I was hearing. No change? No effect after all that poison? After all this time? "What about radiation?"

"Radiation is extremely dangerous for Michael, since he is two years old. It would severely damage his brain. That's not an option here." He sighed. "Go home tonight, and I'll make some phone calls and do further research. I have a colleague that I want to consult with. I'll call you tomorrow with a more definite plan."

The Black Cloud left the room.

I sat holding Michael and rocking back and forth. I had such big hopes this would show some good results, just one little difference, for the better—that was all I needed to hang on. A small glimmer of hope, and Dr. Ebb couldn't deliver.

The walk from the room to the elevator made me feel as if my legs weighed a hundred pounds each, heavy and slow. I dragged my body with every step. I had shrunk to a mere hundred pounds myself, with worry and not eating, yet my body felt like I weighed a thousand pounds. Elise, one of the nurses on Michael's team, escorted us the elevator and pushed the lobby button.

I hugged Elise at the elevator and cried on her shoulder. "I want this to be over."

Once in the car, I called Mark to explain what Dr. Ebb had told us, and cried throughout the short call. He was on his way home and would land later that evening. At home, my mom was with the girls, waiting for Michael and me. She had prepared dinner, and the girls were in bed by the time I got home. She helped me get Michael comfortable and into his crib. As she was leaving to return home to Winthrop, Mark came in the door, exhausted from his trip. I just hugged him as we stood in the front hallway and cried.

That night, I again grabbed my beautiful burgundy Bible and read my healing scriptures aloud, still not sure what I was doing. I finally managed to get myself to sleep.

Cast all your worries upon him because He cares for you"

—2 Peter 5:7

I have strength for everything through him who empowers me.

—Philippians 4:13

CHAPTER 8

Walking the
Journey Together

THE NEXT MORNING, DR. EBB called as promised.

"The next option is a stem cell transplant," he said. "A drug called Thiotepa will be used to wipe out Michael's immune system. His white blood cells will be removed and frozen, Thiotepa administered, and the white blood cells reintroduced."

I knew in my heart how sick and dangerous this procedure was, but I asked questions anyway. "Will this cure Michael?"

"It could help him, but we still have a long way to go."

"What are his chances of surviving this procedure?"

"Well, it is very risky, given the fact that he'll have no immune system. A common cold and he might die. He'll need to be isolated. That is, only the most necessary people in to see him. No one who is sick, everyone must be masked and gowned, head to toe. If someone drops anything on the floor, it must be cleaned before Michael can touch it."

After those two answers, I couldn't handle asking any more questions. The potential answers were too horrible to contemplate.

I almost backed out of this procedure. I actually called Dr. Ebb's office and cancelled the preliminary appointment to meet with him. I just wanted Michael healed and believed in my heart we didn't need this procedure. I convinced myself God would heal him.

Mark, I am sure didn't know what to do. I remember him being supportive of my feelings and faith. He said little, and knew the stem cell transplant had to be done, I guess he allowed me my space in agreeing with him and the doctors.

Two days later, Mark, Michael, and I met with Dr. Ebb at his office. The Black Cloud was now a bit stern with us, but frank. "If you don't have this done, Michael will die. We can make him as comfortable as possible, with morphine, but it won't be long."

That appointment decided Michael's fate, and we started to prepare for the stem cell transplant. Mark, I am sure didn't know what to do.

We had no choice, no other option.

***

It was now July, and transplant day arrived. Everyone at the blood clinic was very nice, but boy, was I angry! I didn't want to be there. I was scared and worried for Michael.

I sat and watched as IVs were inserted into both of Michael's little arms. They removed the blood from one arm, took the white cells out of the removed blood, then returned the red cells back to Michael in his other arm. I was amazed; it was like science fiction. I didn't know they could do such a thing!

It was a long four hours, and I just was not happy to be there or anywhere near a hospital. I should have been happy that something could be done to help my son, but I just couldn't dig that deep. Not that day.

That afternoon we left the hospital clinic and headed back to our second home on Ellison 17, where Elise waited to greet us and make us feel welcomed again. The administration of Thiotepa would start in the morning. Michael and I sat in bed watching TV together, and Mark stopped in after work to bring us food. My wonderful mom was at her post at my house with Jordan and Kaitlin. Pauline and Arlyne helped me maintain some order and normalcy with Jordan and Kaitlin.

After Mark left that evening, I lay in bed with Michael as he fell asleep, my burgundy Bible a comforting weight in my hands. The pages whispered in the cold hospital air as I turned them. I read my thirty-eight scriptures, understanding a little bit more, but more importantly, knowing that they made me feel better, giving me peace and allowing me to let some of my anger go. It also helped me to feel a sense of control when it seemed I had control over nothing.

> *Then He touched their eyes, and said, "Let it be done for you according to your faith." And their eyes were opened. Jesus warned them sternly, "See that no one knows about this".*
>
> *—Matthew 9:29,30*

> *Cast all your worries upon Him because He cares for you.*
> *—1 Peter 5:7*

The next morning, we started the Thiotepa protocol. It was essentially uneventful. Michael would now be in the double-doored room until his white blood count was at a healthy level, which could take up to a month. He would need red blood cells, so I created a list of friends and family with his blood type who had agreed to give blood. We joked that if Michael had a sudden urge for chocolate, he must have gotten my sister-in-law Chrissy's blood, or if he yearned to run a marathon he had gotten my friend Jean's. It was a small way to have lightness and relief in the middle of this dark procedure.

For the first week, Michael was acting and feeling good, and his white counts were slowly rising. But then he starting vomiting and sleeping a lot. He just wasn't himself. The doctors and nurses were sure it was part of the side effects. But it continued, and Michael looked progressively worse. The nurses suspected something was up. Ellen, one of the nurses on Michael's team, agreed that he did not look good, and by the look on her face, I could tell she was seriously concerned.

Ellen informed Dr. Ebb and once he saw Michael he agreed and Dr. Ebb ordered another MRI to see what was going on in Michael's head. Michael was listless, silent, and still vomiting.

Michael and I were alone in his room, waiting to hear when the MRI would be done, about three in the afternoon, and he started to shake.

"Michael, Michael!" I jumped up and called out.

No response. His head was flung back against the pillow, and his eyes rolled back in his head. His arms were stiff and his little hands were closed and turned outward. His legs were stiff and shaking.

I hit the nurse call button and yelled "Help!"

Immediately, Ellen and Elise were in the room. The next thing I knew, the room was in chaos, with doctors, nurses and machines.

"An IV of phenobarbital!" a nurse called.

"IV of valproate," another doctor said.

Then, "Clonazepam."

The doctors, nurses, and machines continued to swirl around Michael as I stood there, helpless. Michael continued seizing on and off. I moved to be by his head, put my cheek to his, and just kept on whispering, "Jesus is with us. He is in you and in me and will get us through this." Oddly, I remained amazingly calm and composed, not hysterical at all.

Eventually Michael was stabilized and moved to Pediatric Intensive Care.

As I waited for the elevator with Dr. Ebb, I was silent and distant.

Dr. Ebb had his hands in his pockets. "Michael has suffered a major seizure." His voice was slow and methodical. "It lasted a long time and had a major impact on Michael's brain."

"What does that mean?"

"We're not sure, in the long- or short-term. We'll just have to wait and see."

"The bigger the battle, the greater the victory" was my reply. *What was I saying? Where did that come from? And where did that calm Jodi come from during Michael's seizure? Who am I?* At the time, I did not even recognize myself,

The elevator finally arrived, and we stepped on. It seemed to take years to get to the Pediatric Intensive Care Unit. I just wanted to be with Michael, to see him and hold his little hand.

Thankfully, Mark was in town, and he met me at the hospital. My dad, Frank, was in the clinic giving blood for Michael. My father hated hospitals, blood, anything medical. But his family was so important to him it overrode any misgivings he felt about medicine. Mark and I fetched my dad and told him what was going on.

Dr. Ebb sat down with all of us in the PICU. In a small, blank room. No pictures on the walls, no color, just a cold, distant linoleum floor. I remember Dr. Ebb looking stern again, and I'd seen this look before and knew what it meant. The small room closed in on me, and I felt trapped once more.

"Michael has fluid in his brain, a condition called hydrocephalus. We need to put in an external drain in his head to relieve the fluid, called a shunt. Michael needs this. Because of his nonexistent immune system, an operation to insert one isn't feasible. So an external drain from his head will drain any fluid that may form on his brain."

"What about later?"

"Once his immune system is able to handle an operation, we can do an internal shunt inside his head to prevent fluid build-up. I'm afraid there's no real good news here."

Again, I felt that we had no choice.

My dad turned to me and simply said, "Josephine, do as the doctors tell you."

Dr. Ebb said Michael's white cells would go up daily, and that when they reached a safe level, the shunt would be inserted. For the time being, Michael remained heavily sedated on morphine and had about twenty tubes, bags, and machines hooked to him. One very painful side effect of Thiotepa is sores in the throat and esophagus. Just swallowing caused Michael excruciating pain. We hoped that a constant morphine drip would help keep him comfortable.

This made it difficult to assess how the seizure had affected Michael. He laid there, his little hands handcuffed to the bed so he couldn't pull out the drain protruding from his head. I would pick eyelashes off his face and collect the hair from his pillow, not able to bear seeing the visual effects of the chemotherapy. I just wanted to climb into the bed with him, help him make sense of the tubes and wiring. An adult would have a hard time with all the treatments; there was no way to explain to this child what was happening to him—and why.

During those days, I sat with my scriptures and read. I was beginning to understand more and more of their wisdom and how it applied to my life. I brought in a tape recorder in the room that played scriptures. The tape never stopped, just got continually flipped from side to side in an attempt to squeeze every bit of peace we could out of the words. A big note was taped on the tape recorder: DO NOT SHUT OFF, per the mother.

Michael had many nurses when he was in the PICU, and Debbie, a large, pretty blonde with a beautiful smile, was the nurse in charge of Michael. She kept that recorder on. She guarded the door, literally. She was a great advocate for us.

One day shortly after Michael arrived (again) at PICU, the neurologists came to examine Michael and she shooed them away.

"No," she said. "He's resting and comfortable, leave him be." They persisted; Debbie didn't back down. They also wanted to lower Michael's morphine dosage to get a more accurate neurological assessment. Knowing how much more pain this would cause Michael, Debbie would not allow it. In time, he could be assessed.

Another time, Michael was awake and feeling a bit better. The nuero team examined Michael, squeaking a green plastic frog in his face. They wanted him to follow the frog with his eyes and not move his head. Whether Michael didn't understand the instructions or simply couldn't do it, we don't know, but after multiple attempts Debbie said, "Enough! You and that darn frog have to leave!"

Michael's care was constant; there was a nurse in the room with Michael and me or Mark almost all the time. Mark and I would take turns at staying at the hospital and going home for some much needed rest. He had over a dozen tubes hanging from a pole beside his bed; to me it looked like a creature looming over him all the time. The tubes were either infusing something into his IV or on tap to do so shortly. I don't know how they kept it all straight, but they did, and they cared for Michael as if he were their own.

I was—am—grateful to Debbie for taking charge and caring so much for us. I certainly couldn't have done it, having no idea what was best for Michael in his tender state. People like Debbie make me believe that through all our life God puts people in our path to help and guide us.

My sister Anne was a nurse at Massachusetts General Hospital and was a huge helper to me. During the many times when Michael was being treated, Anne stopped by his hospital room, bringing us food. If she wasn't working, she made sure a nurse from her floor came by to check on us. She often left me coffee in the morning or a snack in the afternoon. Anne always had my back.

One particular visit when Michael was having surgery and Mark was away on business, Anne called and wanted to come and be with me.

"No, I am fine."

She persevered, asking again and again if I needed anything. My standard answer was always no.

As I look back now, I think that what I really was trying to say is, "I don't know what I need."

But I would often hang up the phone and an hour later, Anne showed up in the hospital room. She came with pancakes; Michael always asked for them after surgery. A salad with chicken came for me, along with a bottle of red wine. I just hugged her and cried!

At that point, I really needed someone but often found it difficult to articulate exactly what I needed. I thank God for Anne, because she always knew exactly what to do. That day, as we ate, the nurses wheeled Michael in and, sure enough, he was looking for pancakes! There were many moments like that. Many times I would come home to dinner cooked, groceries purchased, or Jordan and Kaitlin gone to sleep over at Auntie Anne's house. She was and continues to be a blessing to me.

After two weeks of being in the PICU since the major seizure, Michael's shunt was finally able to be internalized. He had the surgery and was transferred back "home" to Ellison 17. Ellen, Elise, and his entire team of nurses were there to greet us once again. The sores in Michael's throat had begun to heal, and he talked and seemed more like himself.

It was another month, however, before we were able to go home. On a hot August day, we left the hospital, but we were glad for the sun's warmth that felt so good on our bodies. Being able to take Michael outside was a blessing in itself.

All of Michael's muscles had atrophied, and when he sat on my lap I had to support his whole torso with both my hands to keep him upright. Otherwise, he slumped right down. He couldn't walk, his legs were so weak. Physical and occupational therapists came to work with Michael in our home daily. The side effects of the seizure still remained unknown. An MRI showed extensive damage, but the extent to which this would affect Michael remained a mystery.

I was determined that cancer would not drive Michael's life, and neither would that seizure. Michael and I began to go to healing masses at 2:00 p.m. at Our Lady of Perpetual Help in Roxbury, about an hour away. My mom came along too. The services ran about three hours, so I was gone most of the day. Michael didn't seem to mind as he ate, drank, and looked at books throughout the service.

My family, however, was not totally on board with this. They did not have the faith I did and couldn't see the importance of these services. Technically, no it wasn't "safe" to take an immune-suppressed child into public, but Michael's blood counts were checked twice a week, and they were going up. I know that was partly Mark's worry as well.

I never felt like I was putting Michael in a compromised position, and felt very strongly I wanted to do something to help him get better. The doctors never offered us any hope for Michael to survive, so my faith and scripture readings offered me the hope and peace I so desperately needed then. I never thought he would get sick from going to a healing service, and he never did. I would have done anything I believed in to save Michael.

During one part of the service, you were invited to approach the priest, who would lay hands on you to receive healing. Many times I could rest in the Spirit and fall backward. There were catchers to catch you as you fell, helping you gently to the floor. Michael and I would go up to see Father Edward McDonough, and we would fall, Michael in my arms. I would lie on the floor of this old, old church and feel total peace, Michael's head nestled in my neck, breathing so slowly. I have not felt this sense of peace for months. It was amazing; it felt so good I didn't want to get up! We laid there for probably a minute, but it felt like forever comforting and reassuring.

I left the church those days with my head held high, confident and peaceful, carrying Michael. No answers, just peace. I'm still not sure what happened, all I know is that it made me smile, and I was not ever giving up on it. I would get home around 6:00 p.m., just in time to get dinner ready.

Michael always wanted to be carried and often would say "My legs are broken." I know he was weak, but he needed to walk, to use his muscles. When I did carry him, he would glue his right cheek to my cheek, like he was an extension of my body. Sometimes this was frustrating because, as you can imagine, it made it difficult to do anything!

Mom and Arlyne, my mother-in-law, stayed with me when Mark had to travel. They did the laundry and tried to keep up with the house so that I could care for Michael. I would find myself repeating the scriptures, reading them over and over, reciting them in my head as I cared for Michael. It gave me something to think about as I played, read, maneuvered miniature construction equipment, or just watched television with him. *There Goes a Tractor* was his favorite video to watch. I think we watched it a hundred times!

He also loved to go for rides in his carriage to see all the construction vehicles working in our neighborhood as new houses went up. So we would go for a walk, and I would sit on the sidewalk as Michael relaxed in his carriage, watching the backhoe, grader, paver, or whatever construction vehicle happened to be working at the time. He could do this for hours.

I also tried to feed him. He didn't eat much as he had IV food that supplied him with nine hundred calories a day. However, the doctors had explained that he would need to be weaned off of the IV food. His liver function was checked on a weekly basis to ensure it was normal. The IV food was great as it didn't pass through his stomach and made him feel sick; however, it could harm the liver after prolonged use, so I was always trying to get Michael to eat. As we sat and watched the construction vehicles, I fed him small bits of food. And I mean small, half-inch pieces—a cracker, pieces of pizza, French fries, anything Michael considered palatable food. I had to keep a daily diary of food intake.

Once he was taking in a certain amount of calories, I was able to slowly lower the amount of calories he was getting by IV. If he was distracted with the trucks, I could put a piece of food in his mouth, thinking he would chew it, swallow it, and I could record it as eaten! He didn't have much of an appetite; the doctors had warned me that the chemo dulls the taste buds, lending a metallic tinge to everything eaten. No wonder he did not want to eat!

"I want McDonald's," Michael said sometimes. I would immediately change my route, no matter where I was going, find a McDonalds's, order him fries, and sit there as he put them in his mouth and spit them out. McDonald's would never have been an option under normal circumstances, but I was looking for anything high in fat and calories that my son would eat and gain weight. After our walks, I would take him out of the carriage and all the food I thought he had eaten would fall to the ground! It had just plopped onto his lap. I was so disappointed.

Caring for Michael on a daily basis was a big undertaking. There were many, many doctor appointments, visiting nurses, occupational and physical therapy, medications to inventory and supply maintenance.

One night was especially challenging. Michael had been home from the hospital only a few days and was on a steroid called Decadron. Steroids tended to make Michael very indecisive.

"I want to watch *Barney!*" he said. Once *Barney* was in the player, it was no good. "S*esame Street!*" instead.

"I want to go outside."

"I want to go inside."

"I want to eat."

"I don't want to eat!" It was non-stop and incredibly demanding.

I prepared any food he asked for in an effort to boost his weight. He wasn't eating much at all, and still had the IV feeding tube at night. He slept restlessly, which caused sleepless nights for me. Mark always had to get up early for work, so I tended to Michael at night.

One night he needed an antibiotic at 2:00 a.m. that would run through his IV for an hour, then the tube would need to be flushed. So I was up at 1:45 a.m., preparing the medication to be administered for the infusion at 2:00. I gave him the antibiotics, then lie on the floor next to the crib. Once the hour was up, the pump beeped. I was afraid I wouldn't hear it if I went into my room, so I stayed there with him.

Michael persevered through all this restlessly, and I tried to comfort him by rubbing his back, but nothing seemed to really soothe him. I picked him up and rocked him in the rocking chair. I was so scared. Why was he so restless, whimpering? Was the cancer growing inside of him? The doctors had indicated that there was a good chance of this happening.

I tried not to let my thoughts get the best of me. I grabbed my Bible and flashlight. We had flashlights all over Michael's room from the hospital. I sat in the rocking chair with Michael cradled in my arms, two IVs hanging from the crib, my Bible in my left hand, and a flashlight under my chin. I didn't want to turn the light on, but I needed to read God's word. I don't know how long we remained like this, but I do remember Michael eventually settling down, my thoughts and anxiety abating, and a great sense of peace finally settling in. Eventually, I put him in his crib and climbed back into my bed. I thanked God as he had carried me the last few hours with his words and promises. I fell asleep.

I was constantly amazed at all the things that would happen with Michael on a daily basis. I remember Dr. Ebb laying out Michael's protocol—the plan. I love plans. I thrive on order, structure, and planning. However, plans often aren't helpful in the world of a child with a serious illness.

Many times at night Michael would roll around so much that his central line would come out. I would then call Dr. Ebb, and be scheduled for another trip to the clinic. There, Dr.

Dan Doody would surgically insert another line in Michael. This occurred several times. The port was on his left side, then right, then left, then right. I think his port must have been replaced six times.

One day when Michael was about three years old, we went to the clinic to begin a new regimen of chemotherapy. My dad, Frank, was always there, waiting for us. Dad always had a big smile on his face for us. My dad, who usually talks a lot, really didn't say much those times, but I could see it in his eyes. The first time I saw him in the hospital room after Michael was diagnosed, he hugged me and said, "Josephine, I don't understand. This should be me." I guess my father figured he had lived long enough, but he was only seventy at the time.

Occasionally on these visits, we checked in with the nurse to assess Michael's height and weight. This was always very exciting for me, holding my breath while I hoped and prayed that Michael had gained weight. Michael gaining weight! Hoorah! Simple things became such accomplishments with Michael these days.

We then climbed onto the bed, put on the TV, inserted a video about construction, and waited for the nurse to start the chemo. Michael would lie in the bed and watch *There Goes a Tractor* over and over again.

Michael's nurse, Sheila, began to flush the line and start the chemo, but this particular day the line wouldn't cooperate. She just couldn't flush it. Dr. Ebb determined that the line would need to be replaced before Michael could receive chemo, and Michael needed chemo that day. So Michael and I would stay at Massachusetts General Hospital tonight. My dad left to go home to get us clothing and other needs.

Mark was away, and I called him to tell him that Michael needed surgery. Mark was unable to catch a flight home until later that evening. I was so mad!

This is so unfair! I hate this stuff!

I didn't want to stay in the hospital, and I felt alone and very sorry for myself.

I headed into the operating area dressed, as usual, in the blue paper "Smurf" outfit, covered head to toe and carrying Michael, I was numb. They put us in a holding room just outside the operating room. I sat rocking in the chair with Michael in my arms. He drifted off to sleep, and I prayed, "Jesus, I don't like this. I am afraid, and so tired of all that is going on with Michael. I know you can hear me and can help. Please help me."

As I sat there, eyes closed and tears rolling down my face, I felt as if someone came from behind and gave Michael and me a big hug. It was a warm, comforting, and peaceful feeling, lasting only a few seconds. When it was over, the door opened and the operating room nurse announced they were ready for Michael. I handed him over. Tears filled my eyes, but they were not tears of anxiousness but of relief, knowing that Michael would be fine.

As I walked the narrow hallways back to the waiting area alone, hearing only the paper-y sound of my Smurf costume, I felt more peaceful with every step I took. I realized that, in that holding room, rocking Michael, that he would be okay, and we would walk this journey together with Jesus in peace, in confidence that Michael would be just fine.

The oddest thing to me was that I had no answers, nothing had changed, yet I had an unexplainable feeling of peace and comfort. I had no idea what this journey would be with Michael, but somehow, I didn't need to know. For the moment, I felt the peace that I had longed for a very long time.

> *Blessed be the Lord day by day, God, our salvation, who carries us*

> —*Psalm 68:20*

CHAPTER 9

Beginnings and Endings

It was June 10, 1977, and the phone in my house was ringing off the hook. With four teenagers in the house and it being a Friday night, everyone was making plans. My mom always said our house was organized chaos, and this night was a clear example.

My friend Pam had called earlier that day. "My parents are away for the weekend at an Elks Convention and wouldn't be home until Sunday. You know what that means?"

"Party at 1183 Saratoga Street," I said and squealed with delight. Pam had two older brothers, Michael and Mark, so between the three of them, our friends, their friends, and invited friends, we had the ingredients for a great party. I was fourteen, Pam was fifteen, her brother Mark was sixteen, and Michael was eighteen.

The small bathroom was crammed full as my sisters and I got ready that evening. The boombox blared out "Sir Duke" and "Hotel California." Curling irons looped over the counter, and we both had blow dryers going. Once in a while, one of my poor brothers swooped in to quickly dry his own hair, then he was booted out so we girls could continue primping. Pots of makeup, rouge, and eyeshadow were scattered about. I put on my best Vidal Sassoon jeans, checked myself in the mirror, and grinned, full of anticipation about this party.

I'd seen Mark around Winthrop and thought he and his friends were terribly cute. His eyes were breathtaking. Being at a party with older guys was something to look forward to.

I headed to Pam's house in the next town over. As the night progressed, I noticed Pam's brother, Mark, staring at me. He wore white carpenter pants and a royal blue flannel plaid shirt. We flirted, talking and smiling at one another, and Mark eventually invited me to sit on his lap. We looked into each others eyes and kissed! *Wow!* What a feeling!

Mark became my first real boyfriend. I had had boyfriends before, but truly they were more like friends. Mark was very handsome, with beautiful blue eyes and the brightest smile you can imagine. He had awesome brown hair that he wore feathered back. I fell big for Mark, and knew that this was not just a passing thing. Little did I know that this was the beginning of a very long courtship.

We rarely got away with anything. Mark's mom, Arlyne, had the eyes and intuition of a hawk. If one thing was out of place when she returned, she knew it, and would call you out on it. One time a visitor (who wasn't supposed to be in the house at all) had left a watch on her bureau, which was the beginning of a lot of explaining. Michael, Mark, and Pam were grounded for breaking the rules.

That first summer, in '77, Mark went off to track camp for two weeks. He somehow managed to write me a card every day. So every day he was gone, I received a card in the mail, telling me how much he missed me and couldn't wait to see me again. I'm still not sure how he managed that, but I was extremely flattered.

Dating Mark in high school was both difficult and wonderful for both of us. We loved each other, but having the same boyfriend during that time, while developing and figuring myself out made for challenging years. However, we managed to stay together through high school, albeit with a few breakups here and there.

Mark was a partier, and I was the more serious, level-headed one. Mark was a smart guy, but he definitely knew how to have fun. At parties Mark would always be mixing the drinks, "Goombay Smash" or "Sammy's Motion Potion." Growing up, his friends called him Sammy or Sambo. Even today his license plate reads "Sammy," which was his brother Michael's license plate.

Michael was always letting his younger brother Mark take his car, a white Monte Carlo and clean as anything. Michael drove a bus for a living, and we picked him up at work if we used his car that day. Once we pulled up to the bus company, but Mark and I couldn't see Michael, who was usually waiting outside for us. We looked and looked but didn't see him.

"Sambo!" we heard and looked up to find Michael sitting on the roof of one of the buses in the parking lot, shirtless! It was a beautiful day, and he was getting some sun. He jumped down, and off we went!

They were only fifteen months apart, and shared a bedroom until Michael was twenty years old and moved out. I can only imagine what they saw, shared, and talked about together all those years.

The rule was no TV after 11 p.m., so they rigged up some kind of device that shut off the TV when their bedroom door was opened. "You must be hearing something outside, it's not us," they would say to their puzzled parents.

Michael always made me laugh with jokes that I never truly understood. He used to pick up my hair and ask, "Are you blond under there?" He was full of life, and whenever I would see him, he would pick me up twirl me around saying, "You're so light," and "Jodi babeeeeeee." Easygoing without a care in the world, Kaitlin reminds me of him.

❧

By Labor Day weekend of 1982, Mark and I had been dating for five years. I was nineteen, and he was twenty-two. We were very serious about each other.

At the time, Michael had just broken up with a longtime girlfriend. She wanted to settle down, looking for some kind of a commitment, but he still thought there was a lot of fun to be had as a single guy; after all, he was only twenty-two.

A female friend asked him to a wedding. He liked her but just as a friend. I had several conversations with him about whether or not he should attend the wedding. He was very apprehensive; he didn't want his friend to get the wrong idea, but he knew it would be a good time. After much hesitation, he decided to attend the wedding.

Mark and I were away that weekend at my family's house in New Hampshire, it being the last weekend of summer. It was about 2 a.m., and we had just gotten back after being out partying with cousins when the phone rang. This couldn't be good, who calls at that hour?

My father picked it up. "Mark's father is on the phone," he said and handed it to Mark.

Mark took the heavy black hand piece; I still remember that awful blue "pleather" chair with the nail heads on it. His head was down and he just listened. When he hung up, the look of despair and shock on his face made my chest go tight.

"There's been an accident. We have to get to Lynn Hospital right away."

Mark and I left as quickly as possible, and headed out for the three-hour drive to Lynn hospital. Mark was in no shape to drive, so I drove as he laid his head on my lap in the front seat. My mind was racing. What would we find when we get to the hospital? Accident? Car accident? They didn't elaborate. My stomach did somersaults, and my shoulders and neck were as stiff as cement. I clutched the steering wheel as I drove down I-95, white knuckled. I just looked straight ahead and prayed.

We didn't say a word; there were none to say.

All I could do was recite the Hail Mary and Our Father. As we finally approached the hospital, Mark awoke. We ran inside and looked frantically for Arlyne and Stan. We were directed to the third floor, and we made our way up.

Arlyne, Pam, and Stan were there, the women trembling and crying. "Michael was shot," Stan said.

Shot? I am not hearing this! I thought it was a car accident. He was at a wedding!

Mark grabbed his family, and they all stood there in a family hug that lasted a very long time. I was crying, in shock and disbelief.

Apparently, there had been a party in a hotel room after the wedding, and a guest had bragged about a gun. He went out to his car and brought the gun to the party. The gun discharged and hit Michael in the head. Michael now lay in a coma with a bullet lodged in his skull and on a respirator, barely alive. The doctors explained that only time would tell if the bullet could be safely removed.

We held vigil at Michael's bedside from that day on. The family was always together, talking, praying, standing at Michael's side.

A week later, the doctors explained that the bullet had moved and was inoperable. Michael had no brain activity. He was in a vegetative state; only the respirator was keeping him alive. He wouldn't have wanted to live like this, so the family decided not to keep him on the respirator. He died on September 11, 1982.

It was my first experience with death, especially of someone of such a young age.

The pain and heartache was unbearable for Mark and his family. I don't think it is something you ever get over. The years have dulled the pain and heartache, but it is still there, just duller. I think when we have such tragedies in our lives, we go back to what we know helps us to cope, to heal.

The pain and heartache was a lesson we needed to learn then, to help us cope now.

Fear not, I am with you; be not dismayed; I am your God

—Isaiah 41:10

CHAPTER 10

Running for Life

IN 2000 MICHAEL'S CARE HAD settled into a more "normal" routine, if caring for a deathly ill child can ever be called normal. But we had a schedule and a plan for treatment so we all soldiered on. The girls were growing up, Michael was gaining weight and eating, and I was bolstered by his progress and my faith. So when the MGH team approached us about running the Boston Marathon in honor of Michael for brain tumor research, I thought, *That is just what Mark needs!* Mark had been an accomplished cross-country runner in high school, winning many awards and scholarships.

The Boston Marathon starts in Hopkinton and finishes on Boylston Street in downtown Boston, 26.2 miles of a series of hills, very difficult hills. One section is called "heartbreak hill," and it's really a series of six hills at about the twenty-mile marker. At this point in the marathon, it seems doable. It the hardest six miles anyone could ever run. Your legs start to cramp up, blisters form on your feet, your body is aching all over, and all you want to do is stop. Things start happening to your body that you never thought would happen. The last thing you want to do is run six more miles up a hill!

Prepping for the marathon took a lot of training. For Mark, it started in December and lasted until the day of the marathon, held on April 17. Training for the marathon on the East Coast was a challenge in itself. There were many cold, snowy, rainy, nine-degree days where Mark had a ten- or fifteen-mile run ahead of him. He always got it done. Mark took the training very seriously; he put his heart and soul into running this marathon. He ran with the MGH team on the weekends in Boston and come home and took a jacuzzi with Michael to ease his tired muscles. Weekends were dedicated to running and resting. He didn't drink alcohol and followed a strict eating regiment.

For Mark, this was a way to regain a certain amount of control over things that he had had no control over. Most weekends, Mark set out for his fifteen-mile run, and the kids and I piled into the Caravan and drove down the road to meet Mark at designated streets. We made sure he had plenty of water and GU, a gel pack that kept athletes fueled during long competitions, whatever he needed. It was definitely something good for our family; we needed to focus on something good in our lives. I was happy to support him, and I understood the toll training for a marathon took on his body. The hard work and dedication that was such a positive force for Mark spilled over and helped the rest of the family too.

Being part of the MGH marathon team also meant fundraising. Mark was paired up with Michael, running in honor of him. He pledged to raise two thousand dollars as part of his commitment to the team. Ninety-five percent of all the funds raised from the MGH marathon team go to research. The fundraising part was my job. I focused on getting the media to cover Mark's marathon story. Channel 5 in Boston did a beautiful story on Mark and Michael, and ran it several times prior to the race. They also aired our address for people to mail donations. It was overwhelming!

We began to receive a steady stream of letters, stories, and donations in the daily mail, one of the rare times it was exciting to get the mail every day. Many people wrote about how inspiring our story was and how they changed their own lives based on hearing our story. We even received a letter from a dad who was incarcerated and who said his goal to be a better dad.

We also had Joe Fitzgerald from *the Boston Herald* write a story about our family, and Mark running the Boston Marathon. That article prompted more letters, cards, stories, and donations.

On April 9 of 2000, we organized a "Michael Sampson Day" at Richardson's Dairy Farm in Middleton, a local outdoor entertainment center with ice cream, mini golf, batting cages, driving range, and a farm. We had mini golf contests, face painting, a band, raffle tickets, and ice cream. We had signs up all over town, urging merchants and residents to support our efforts by volunteering, donating, anything to help. With all the fundraising, we raised our thirty-five thousand dollars that year!

The week before Michael Sampson Day, my doorbell rang. Outside stood two Masconomet High School baseball players, dressed in uniform.

"This is for Michael," they said and handed me a package.

"Thank you," I replied, puzzled and intrigued.

When I opened the box, I started to cry—it was a high school baseball uniform. Included in the box was a note from baseball coach Peter Delani:

> *Dear Sampson family,*
>
> *When Michael gets to Masco I would love to coach him. He already has a spot on the baseball team.*

As I took the uniform out of the package, I couldn't help but notice how big it was. Michael was only four at the time, and the thought of him being old enough to wear this uniform, surviving this whole cancer ordeal and making it to Masco was a dream I forced myself to believe in as I hugged that uniform and tears rolled down my cheeks.

᪥

On April 17th, on the marathon route, the MGH team camped out at the twenty-mile mark to encourage team runners. Mark stopped briefly for a picture with Michael but had to keep running so he wouldn't get cramps in his legs. He looked amazing, so strong, but I wasn't sure what shape he would be in after twenty-six miles. He had mentally run the marathon countless times in his head and was convinced on a time of 3:41, and he achieved it!

Our whole family was there—Jordan, Kaitlin, my parents, Mark's parents and, of course, Michael. It was a cool day, in the fifties, with the sun shining. Good marathon weather.

Michael I don't think grasped all that was going on. He was excited to see Mark as he came by us at mile twenty.

"How does he look?" I asked Michael.

"He was all sweaty," Michael said. This was probably the first time Michael actually looked good. He looked healthier, had color in his cheeks, and actually had cheeks! His hair had grown back, and he was feeling good that day. He had a a denim quilted jacket with Mickey Mouse embroidered on the front. For most of the day, he sat on my shoulders as we watched the runners pass us by, waiting for Mark.

It was the first time in a long time that I felt a bit of control over my life. Once we greeted Mark at the twenty-mile marker, we piled into the car to meet him at the finish line. As Mark crossed the finish line at his expected time of

3:41, the whole family was there to greet, hug, squeeze, and congratulate him! We had come together as a family set out to do something great, and we did!

For once, I felt part of the "real world" again, happy to be Jodi again. That marathon was a great day for Mark and the Sampson family.

> *He said to them, "I will come and cure him".*
>
> —*Matthew 8:7*

CHAPTER 11

What Is Normal?

By 2001 MICHAEL WAS AGE five, and we were all trying to live a normal life with normal routines. He attended preschool at Fuller Meadow five mornings a week. Most parents drove up to the front, dropped their children off, and waved good-bye as the kids ran to greet friends. This was not the case for Michael and me. I too would pull up in front but instead put the car in park and take the keys out of the ignition. Michael would cling to me as I picked him up out of the car and carried him down the hallway covered with paintings and crafts, the smell of glue and paper in the air. I remember this walk too well; I did it five days a week. While many parents may have looked at me, questioning my judgments, this was normal for me. And while I may have walked away crying each morning, I was happy that I was walking down the halls of Michael's school rather than down the halls of the hospital. This, to me, meant normal was near.

Many mornings I tried to leave him at the front door, but Michael's left cheek was glued to my right. When I tried to put him down, he lifted up his legs, refusing to put down the landing gear. So I would simply walk Michael to his classroom, where the aide, Mrs. Cerullo, peeled him off me as he sobbed. I quickly turned away and walked briskly back down the hall. I do this both for him and for me.

Every day I walked with him to the classroom. I was told he was fine and cooperative once I was gone; it was the initial separation that riled him. Eventually I began to put him down and walk with him to the classroom, and thought, *Progress.* By January of 2002, I could leave him at the door like all the other moms, and wave good-bye. He was smiling and happy as he faded into the distance.

That cold day in January, I started to cry.

I stood there for a few moments and stared at the closed doors. I had thought that life with Michael would always be about challenges, perseverance, never giving up, hope, faith, joy, sadness, with every other emotion mixed in. I managed to stop crying, caught my breath, and headed to the gym. I had time to refocus my attention to the exercises I ripped out of a fitness magazine that I wanted to try. I was free for four hours to exercise, grocery shop, clean, and get back to the school by 12:30.

As time went by, Michael settled into a chemo schedule that fits into his new life: Mondays from 1:00 to 4:00, six weeks on, two weeks off. Over time I convinced Dr. Ebb that

I knew enough about Michael's chemo to allow him to take it at home with the help of a visiting nurse, an arrangement that would be better for me and for Michael.

Over the past three years, I had gained Dr. Ebb's trust and faith. He knew that I would always do what was best for Michael. Dr. Ebb was great like that, a very reasonable man. Many times I called him to express my concern at the way Michael was behaving, or to report that he was vomiting more than was normal. Or I would simply say, "I'm coming in," and we would trek to the hospital clinic. I only visited MGH when absolutely necessary.

Dr. Ebb turned out to be a blessing to me and my family. He was a very professional and smart doctor, yet he totally understood the "whole picture" and how Michael's illness affected the whole family. He was very straightforward with me, clear and truthful, yet had compassion and Michael's best interest at heart. I could discuss my concerns about Michael, and he was always ready with an answer.

If he needed to consult with other doctors, he would get back to me right away. Michael's health and the complexity of his disease made his care very complicated, necessitating the need for a team of many different doctors to weigh in on Michael's case at any given time. He had an oncologist, neurologist, neurosurgeon, medical surgeon, neuro ophthalmologist, psychologist, audiologist, endocrinologist, seizure doctor, and on and on. Any decisions about Michael's care were made by his team, some of the most respected doctors in their fields. Most of his doctors had appeared on medical magazine covers and ranked number one in the world. There were dignitaries, foreign leaders, and actors who flew from all around the world to be seen by these doctors. I had them all at my disposal, anytime, and only twenty miles away from my home. How blessed I felt!

I consider Dr. Ebb both Michael's doctor and a trusted friend. If I wanted to skip a chemotherapy appointment because we had a family obligation, or if we needed to postpone a chemotherapy appointment because of vacation, Dr. Ebb was willing to help us out. "In the long run," he said, "it won't do any harm." On several occasions, when I did end up at the MGH emergency room, Dr. Ebb organized and made the ER aware that I was coming in with Michael. I found him there, talking with the ER doctors and telling them Michael's history and what needed to be done to assess his situation.

One time in '02, during a visit to the emergency room, Dr. Ebb quickly got the doctors to attend to Michael when he was in particular distress, and Michael was diagnosed in no time. His Dilantin level, an anti-seizure medication, was low. The daily dosage was based on body mass, and since Michael had grown, his levels were now too low to effectively prevent seizures. Once we administered him the correct dosage of Dilantin, Michael was back to himself. We were then on our way as Dr. Ebb escorted us to the main entrance of the hospital. He truly cared. He always returned my phone calls, and even gave me his cell phone number!

When I would speak of my faith or spirituality or say something like, "God will get Michael through this," or "God has a great plan for Michael's life," Dr. Ebb would just look at me and smile. Sometimes he would say, "Whatever you are doing is working, keep doing it." I never expected him or anyone to understand my faith, yet he definitely respected it!

Sherry was Michael's chemo/IV nurse who came to the house on Mondays. She was tall and attractive, with a long blond ponytail. In her mid-thirties, she was engaging, but not too chatty. In her bright-colored scrubs, she wore a cheerful smile while carefully observing Michael. Many times after she hooked him up with his chemotherapy, he sat at the kitchen table and ate.

"I've never seen anyone eat so much through chemo," she said, amazed. She was also pleased with his labs. She always looked over the reports before she started his chemo. "Usually the blood cell count goes down, but Michael's stays within in the normal range."

Sometimes when I came back into the kitchen, Sherry would just be staring at Michael, maybe in amazement or observation, I don't know. It was a great sight to me!

We arrived home from school at 12:40, and I would bring up the box and IV pole from the basement. Sherry rang the doorbell at 12:50. Papa (my dad) came through the door at 12:55. By 1:00, Michael was all hooked up to an IV and getting his chemotherapy, Irinotecan, sitting with Papa and Sherry to eat lunch, chat, or watch television. This was just a great sight—finally, Michael was eating! I had to appreciate the moments for what they were. I had to forget for the moment that he had an IV in his arm and poisonous liquid coursing through his veins. He was eating, swallowing, and enjoying food once again!

It had been just over a year since we had managed to wean Michael off of the IV food. That process started when Dr. Ebb told us that Michael's kidney functions were starting to show overuse. "If Michael doesn't start eating, we'll have to stop the IV food and start with a feeding tube."

I couldn't believe what I was hearing: more changes, more decisions, more medical stuff that just turned my stomach. I was determined to get Michael to eat, and by lowering his IV food by two hundred calories at a time, we started to see Michael regain an appetite.

Slowly over that year, Michael began eating regular food, and we drop-kicked the IV for food. One of the happiest days I remember was packing up the IV pole, the tubes, the syringes, the alcohol wipes, the heparin and taking it to the post office for that last time! Michael and I made many trips to the post office to drop off packages, but that day was such a great experience.

We walked up to the counter and I slammed that box down.

Phil, the mail worker, asked, "Wow, what was that for?" He knew all about Michael.

I explained what was in the box and that we were sending it all back.

"Well, in that case," Phil said, and he picked up the box and slammed it on the counter again!

Michael, Phil, and I all laughed and gladly stamped that box back to where it belonged. Michael and I went out to celebrate by eating. His choice, of course: Friendly's!

Eating in the Sampson home took on a new meaning! I loved to cook, but more importantly, I loved to see my family eat my food. I get such joy out of the smells, talk, and laughter that always seemed to emerge from the kitchen table. Many days I would just sit and watch Michael chew, eat, swallow, and enjoy the food and not spit it out. I guess my Italian heritage was kicking in. If you ate, you were happy; if you did not eat, well, something was wrong! I realized as I sat and watched Michael eat, it would be the small things that other parents take for granted, but I relished what I saw that day.

We didn't abuse our bodies, but I felt there was room for improvement. We needed to incorporate more whole foods, fruits, and vegetables. Once I started to read labels, I realized that I had no clue as to what we were eating, and how that affected our bodies. An apple is an apple, nothing hidden there. However, do you buy organic, or can you get away with the regular fruits and veggies?

I started to buy only organic, but feeding five people on a one-earner family income became challenging. I left the organic grocery store with two bags of fruits, veggies, and whole grains, having spent eighty dollars. When you pay two dollars for an apple, you expect your children to eat the entire apple. My trips became less frequent to the organic store, and more frequent to the stores that saved me money.

Plus, we had the juicer. I juiced carrots, celery, beets, apples, pears, radishes, kale, you name it. If I could fit it in my juicer, it got juiced! I've now realized I can eat healthy, buy regular groceries, and not go broke doing it!

It was challenging, but we all eat more whole foods, less carbs, and fewer foods that are loaded with fat and sugar. Mark and I together have become much more educated about foods and have fun cooking new recipes and passing all we have learned onto the kids. After a cancer diagnosis, I wanted to do everything in our power to stay healthy and prevent any reoccurrences. Food was the one thing I could control, and since I love to cook, it was a great match.

During the chemo sessions, as Michael sat with Sherry and Dad, I tried to get all the household tasks done. I ran up and down the stairs doing laundry, making beds, answering the phone, paying bills, all those things that take time—but I had so little time to get done. I used the time Michael was in school for "me time," a workout at the gym, getting my hair cut or an occasional facial or massage, meditation, much-needed quiet time, or just running errands and grocery shopping. I realized how important my health and mind needed to be to care for Michael and meet all the challenges that will come our way with a child like him. So I was diligent to take care of myself, mind, body, and soul!

I used the time my dad was at the house to get house stuff done, and was very appreciative. I checked on everyone, made sure everything was running smoothly, but it always was, and by 4:00 Sherry was all packed up and out the door, followed by Papa. As soon as they left, I packed up my IV pole and medical box, and down to the cellar it went. I still had a pantry with medical supplies, but I just couldn't bear to look at the IV apparatus a moment longer. I knew it was helping Michael and saving his life, so a part of me was grateful. But I also hated it! I was way too familiar with the other side of chemo, chemo that doesn't work!

There were two other children who had brain tumors who Michael and I had become friendly with during our trips to the hospital for chemo: Matthew and Tammy. We were all on the same chemo schedule, and talked often. We always sought each other out, and felt scared when those familiar faces didn't show up.

During one day visit in 2000, Sheila, the nurse, had just leaned over Michael, prepping his line for the chemo.

"Where's Matthew?" I asked.

"He died," she answered.

I plopped down on the chair, shocked and nauseated. Died? How could that be? We just saw him last week! I started to cry. Sheila continued with Michael's chemo and put her hand on my back. We didn't speak anymore.

Andrew was a seven-year-old Hispanic boy, and his mom, dad, and sister, Debbie, came to the hospital on his chemo days, which were the same days as Michael's. Debbie was a bubbly three- or four-year-old who bounced around the office and visited all the patients as they endured chemo. She was naturally happy and always made Michael laugh. She lightened the mood of the entire office. I often talked to her, and she would tell me about her life and all about Andrew. Her parents didn't speak English well, and they just always looked worried and concerned.

One day, as I was waiting during Michael's chemo, Debbie came skipping in and singing, "Andrew is getting his line out! Andrew is getting his line out!" This, of course, meant that Andrew was done with chemo and was getting his central line out. He was in remission and on his way to enjoying life! I was so happy for Andrew, Debbie, and her parents, but felt sorry for Michael and me.

It had been four years since Michael had been diagnosed, and I wanted Michael to be in remission too! We all hugged.

"We wish you well," I said. "I hope we never see you again!" They knew what we meant.

I sat back in my chair and waited for Michael to be done with his chemo. I couldn't help but think, *I want to be them! God, why? Why can't Michael and I be like Andrew and his family and walk out of this hospital today, cancer-free, no central line, and in remission!* I was mad and tired and envious, all those emotions building up inside me.

About nine months later, I got a dose of *thank God that he does not answer all our prayers.* My mom and dad had come to my house for dinner on a Sunday afternoon. My mom handed me a newspaper clipping from the *the Boston Globe*. She usually shares a recipe of some kind, or news on the Catholic Church, or a doctor at MGH lobbying for funding for brain tumor research.

She handed me the newspaper clipping from the obituary section. She said to me, "Isn't that the same boy that was in the hospital with Michael?" I looked at the picture, and the name: Andrew. I couldn't believe it! I dropped to the chair and started to cry. I instantly recalled wanting Michael to be Andrew that day at MGH, as Debbie skipped around the office, mad at God that it wasn't Michael's turn to be in remission!

I went upstairs and got on my knees and cried uncontrollably. I'm not sure how long I remained there, reduced to a puddle of tears and on my knees. I cried for me, feeling so terrible about wishing to be someone else, crying for Michael that it wasn't over, and crying for Andrew and his family. They were all so happy; the parents' faces had finally looked happy, not that concerned worried usual look on their faces.

I learned so much that day. Sometimes we don't get our prayers answered because they aren't as clear-cut as they seem. I guess I just wanted out, out of MGH, out of all the doctors, out of everything related to cancer! I had so wanted my prayers answered that day. Thank God he does not answer all our prayers.

I walked out of the hospital that day, holding Michael, clinging to him and crying and feeling grateful to be walking out of the hospital, guilty that Michael survived, mad that children had to die. So many emotions, numbing thoughts. With that experience in the back of my mind, I constantly needed to keep my anger and hatred of chemo in perspective.

Those days in 2002 were happier for all of us. Often, Michael and I headed for the pool, where we both swam so that Michael could get some much-needed exercise. We sat on a noodle together and pretended we were riding a bike, peddling faster and faster all around the pool. Then I'd have Michael turn onto his stomach, holding him by his waist, and help him swim the freestyle, constantly repeating, "Reach and pull, reach and pull," while he practiced his swimming strokes. He enjoyed this so much!

I was happy to finally bring him to someplace other than the hospital, to allow him to be a normal five-year-old boy. Even though I didn't really like pools, it didn't matter to me. Michael was happy and smiling, and I enjoyed watching him be happy. We would spend a half-hour in the pool, then head back home. Since I disliked the smell of chlorine, I would immediately shower to rid myself of that awful smell, and start dinner.

Life was beginning to be manageable now, and somewhat normal. Other than chemo on Mondays, and weekly visits to MGH for checkups and MRIs, we carried on like a regular family.

Life was getting to be good.

Miracle Child

There sits a boy in a white wicker chair
Eyes like the ocean you would have to stop and stare
Candy in his hands, he is happy as can be
Something he fighting inside, no one can see
In June we got the news that dropped our jaws
The doctors said he wouldn't make it to see Santa Clause
With the smile on his face, it appears nothing is wrong
As each day goes by my mom and dad stay strong
Dad participates in the famous Boston April race
He raised money for the cause with style and grace
Mom stayed at the hospital day and day out
With lots of things on her mind but especially not doubt
It was a time so scary and horrifying,
worry upon worry piled
But he survived the horrible time, and
they called him the Miracle Child.

Written by:
Kaitlin Sampson
2001

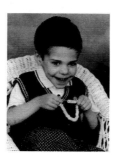

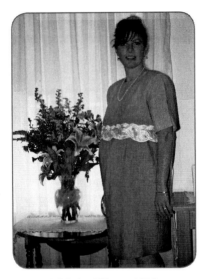

Me pregnant with Michael Easter 1996, one month to go

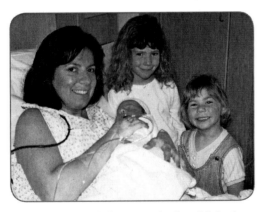

At the hospital after giving birth to Michael,
with Jordan & Kaitlin—May 1996

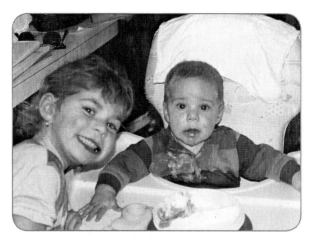

Michael and Kaitlin—6 months old eating peas

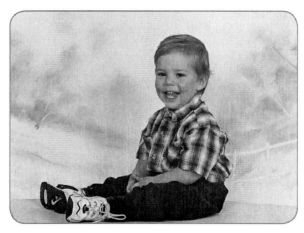

Michael—April 1997—11 months old

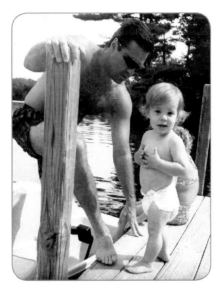

Michael at Lake Winnepausake 1997—1 year old

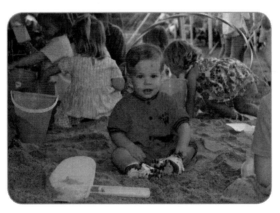

Meditech Outing—Michael September 1997—15 months old

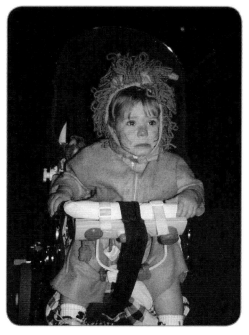

Halloween—October 1997—Michael was mad because I put
him in the carriage and he wanted to run. 16 months old

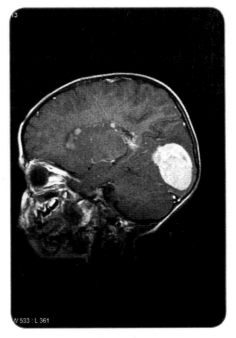

Initial MRI to diagnose brain tumor 1998

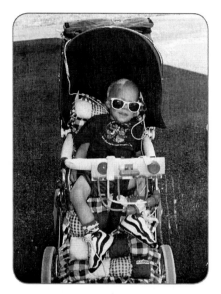

Michael after first surgery May 1998

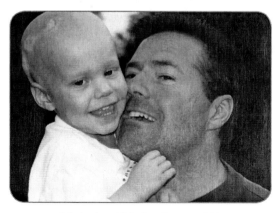

Michael and Mark—August 1998

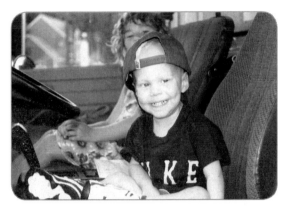

Michael looking happy—September-1998

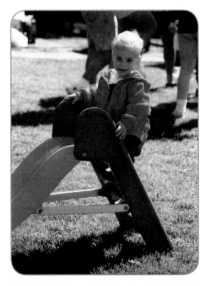

Michael—in our backyard—April 1999

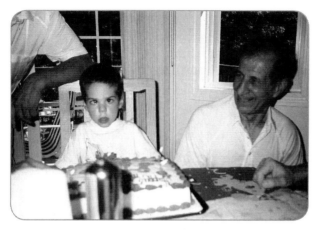

Michael's 3rd birthday—May 1999 with his "googly eyes"

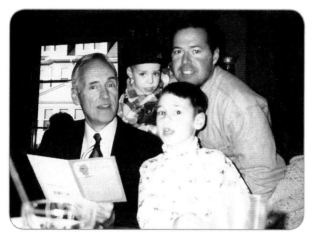

Grampie, Michael, Mark and Sam—November 1999

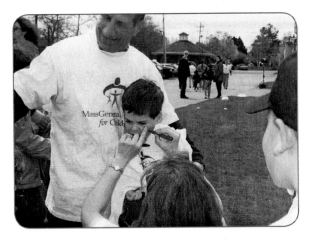

Michael and Papa—Michael Sampson Day—2000

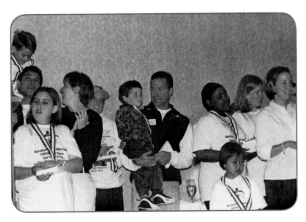

Boston Marathon photos—Michael and Mark
at the MGH pasta dinner—2000

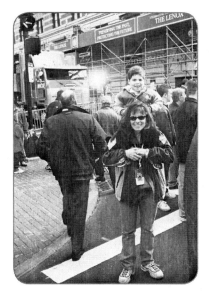

Michael and I at the Boston Marathon 2000

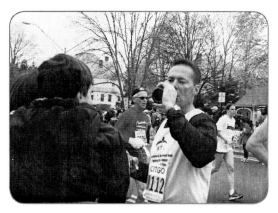

Mark at mile 20 of the marathon

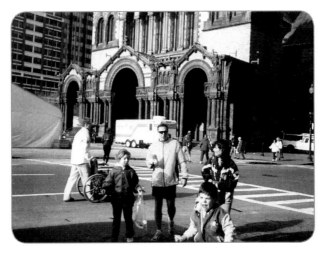

Kaitlin, Mark, Michael & I at the end of the Boston Marathon

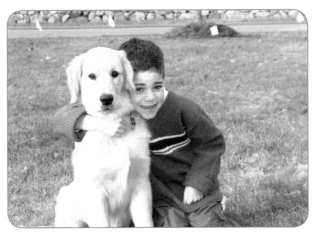

Michael and Boomer—2001

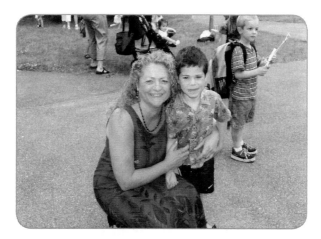

Michael with pre-school teacher Mrs. "R"

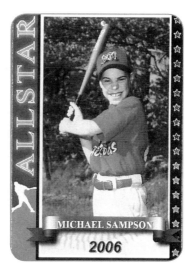

Michael baseball card—"Muckdogs"-2006

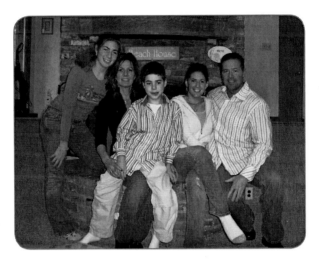

Christmas 2006

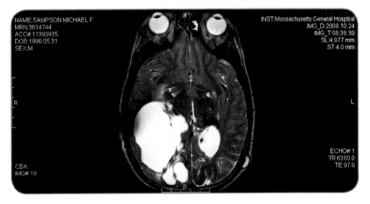

blocked shunt 2008

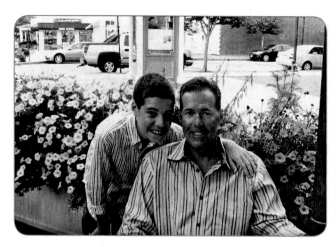

Mark and Michael at the cape 2009

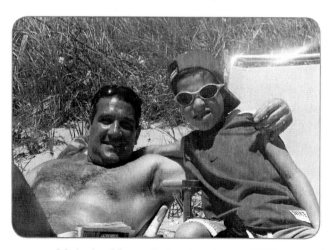

Michael and Joe on the beach at the cape 2008

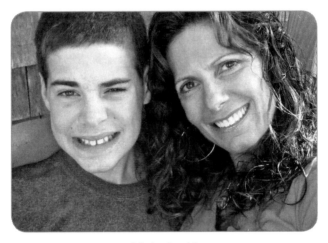

Michael and I

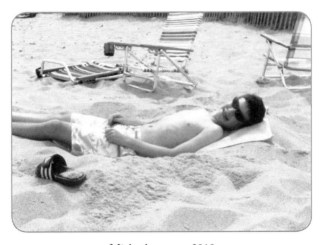

Michael summer 2010

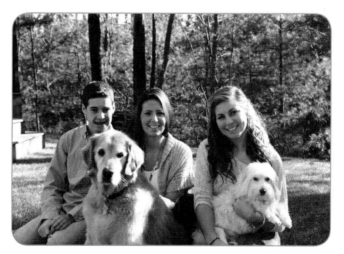

Christmas 2011

CHAPTER 12

The Colors of our Lives

In 2003 Jordan was ten years old, and Kaitlin eight. Jordan had curly blond hair, like Shirley Temple, and she had my face and brown eyes. She was long and lanky then, considerably taller than Michael. Most nights I went in to cuddle with the girls before they fell asleep.

One night, as I lay in Jordan's bed, she asked me, "Mom, is Michael going to die? I hear people dying of cancer often and it scares me."

"I believe Michael will live a long life, that God has a plan for him that we just don't know yet. We need to have faith and trust, even during the unknown." We had similar conversations as time went by, and I think Jordan came to rely on them to calm her fears. She also witnessed in me a confidence. Even if she didn't yet have my faith in God, she had faith in me.

A bit younger, Kaitlin had thin light brown hair and blue eyes. Hers was a more athletic build, stronger-looking and muscular. Kaitlin's conversations at night were a bit different, as different as the two girls were. She didn't ask many questions, but one night she shocked me.

"I know how Michael got cancer, and it's my fault."

"What do you mean? Of course it's not your fault, it's no one's fault."

"I saw Michael eat a green crayon once, and I thought it was funny. So I didn't stop him. And green crayons cause cancer!"

"Oh, precious," I said and laughed gently. "Yes, you should have stopped Michael from eating the green crayon, but no, it had nothing to do with him getting cancer. Really." I got a good laugh out of this, but Kaitlin wasn't laughing. I used these times as an opportunity to talk about the food we eat, the environment in which we live, and all the things I think can contribute to a cancer diagnosis, how we need to take care of this world by recycling, and do our part to preserve it.

Later that week, the double doors of scanner number two slowly opened, and seven-year-old Michael was wheeled out. Phase one of the waiting was over. He was wheeled to a day recovery room, warm blankets wrapped all around him. As always, when I walked into the recovery room, I kept my head down. I didn't want to see anything. No machines, no IVs, no drip lines. Michael was wheeled into his cubby.

I kissed his cheek. "Hi, Michael." No response.

He was snoozing comfortably, so phase two of waiting began. Mark and I sat patiently beside his bed, not talking much, just sitting. I was cold, and the nurse brought me a warm blanket too. The walls were grayish-green.

Who picked out these colors? So dull, so depressing. And the curtain they swiftly whipped around us was a dull blue, very pale, and supposedly for "privacy." You could hear everything in the recovery room. Sounds still permeated: kids crying, parents looking for a nurse, yet others looking for something to eat or help going to the bathroom.

Patience was in full swing, and we continued to sit and wait. We called Michael's name again, to no response. Life was about waiting, and waiting patiently. I had come to be a more patient person. If that was part of the test, then I think I passed.

All the monitors were still on Michael, and Bob, the nurse, watched over him. I thanked God that in a few short hours, we would be going home. Many people here wouldn't. I am grateful.

We had an appointment in three weeks to see Dr. Ebb, so for three weeks anyway, Michael will not be back to MGH. Michael slowly opened his eyes. We now had one foot out the door.

A routine MRI is just that, routine, nothing special, just a basic look around to make sure everything is as it should be. But Michael's MRIs were far from routine. They included "contrast," which involved a dye being injected through the IV to highlight tumors and scar tissue, clearly identifying anything out of the ordinary. Ever since the first MRI after Michael's initial chemo, everything had been stable, and he was acting, growing, and eating as a normal child.

I just assumed Dr. Ebb would call us that evening with his usual speech: "Everything is stable, there is still evidence of cancer cells; we can't determine if they are alive or dead, so we will continue with Michael's current chemo protocol." I had come to be okay with that call. I wanted it all gone, completely clear, a miracle! I hoped and prayed for that phone call, but for now I waited.

Dr. Ebb did call us at home later that evening, but with a different speech, and not the one I prayed and hoped for.

"This morning's MRI looks different," he said. "Michael's cancer is growing."

I felt like Mike Tyson had just punched me in the stomach. This couldn't be!

"But he's going to school and acting fine, no vomiting, no neurological signs of anything wrong!"

"We've got you an appointment to see Dr. Tarbell in the morning."

I struggled with the news. More importantly, my head was trying to listen to Dr. Ebb to understand everything he was saying, while at the same time my heart and gut said, "No. He is fine. This is wrong!"

I shook my head as I hung up the phone. "This just feels wrong to me," I said.

"Let's just go to the meeting," Mark said, "and hear what they have to say. We don't have to decide anything right now."

The next morning, along with Dr. Ebb, we met with Dr. Tarbell to discuss the new plan of action for Michael. Tarbell was the head of pediatric radiation at MGH, world-renowned, very smart, and well-respected in the medical community. I hated her!

Dr. Tarbell was an attractive, tall, slender woman with brownish-blond hair to her shoulders, a cute updated hairstyle, and wore a white lab coat. Not really a woman you would naturally hate. I didn't hate her, of course; I hated what she was going to say and why she was in my life. I am sure that if I met her socially, I would think she was a very nice woman—and she was. I just didn't want to see her and talk about any plan for Michael; I knew it wasn't going to be good.

We all viewed the new MRI together. The contrast clearly showed an increase in the cancer compared to the previous one. The doctors were somber, quiet, and seemed nervous as the four of us sat in a small closed-door room.

"This time, radiation is our only option to save Michel's life," Dr. Ebb started. "The chemotherapy we're currently doing isn't working."

"Aren't there alternatives?" Mark asked them. "Other chemos or trials?"

"I'm going to look into other chemotherapies, but most are in phase one clinical trials, with no solid results. I wouldn't be too hopeful that anything will come of them."

"But radiation will damage his brain, right?"

"At this point in time, we need to focus on saving his life first," Dr. Ebb replied. "We can deal with the consequences later."

Dr. Tarbell spoke up, "There's no other option available. Radiation is the only possible chance to save Michael's life."

Radiation for Michael, or any child so young, is devastating, both physically and mentally. Radiation would damage so much of his brain that he may not be able to function completely on his own.

I was shaking and crying, and in the midst of my tears, my heart just spoke, and out of my mouth I spoke these words, "No, Michael will outlive all the people in this room. I don't know how, I don't know when, I don't know why. I simply feel in my heart and gut that this is not right, something is not right."

There was an eerie silence in the room—no one spoke, no one moved, we all just sat there. I couldn't believe I had said what I was feeling, and I knew it would not be received very well. How could it? I probably sounded like a crazy woman, a mother who just couldn't grasp the truth—disillusioned, scared. As we sat there in silence, I saw a small tear run down Dr. Tarbell's left cheek. Was she crying for me, or for Michael? Probably both.

Dr. Ebb, very slowly and methodically, took Mark and I through the MRI scan once more. I understood it, I saw the difference, I saw what everyone else saw. I just felt like someone was screaming to my heart, and I can't explain how or why I said what I said. It's just a knowing. I felt God was speaking to my heart—no answers, no explanation, just letting me know that this was not right. How could I explain that to Dr. Ebb, Dr. Tarbell, and Mark? I guess I wasn't supposed to explain it, just ride it out, stay focused, and pray.

After the meeting, Mark and I very slowly walked to the exit of MGH. I didn't notice anyone or anything. We just walked, not saying a word. What would we say to one another? Words seemed trivial. Michael had come so far, and we were starting to be a normal family again. Beaten up and overwhelmed, we stood outside the hospital parking lot, hugging each other silently. Then Mark went to work. I'm not sure how he did that, but I'm grateful that he was able as we relied too heavily on his salary and health insurance.

My mom was home with Michael, so I felt like I had the time to stop and think. I just could not walk into my house and tell my mom what I'd heard. I wasn't ready, I couldn't get those words out of my mouth: "The cancer has grown."

Before I went home, I stopped in Wakefield at Lake Quannapowitt. I pulled into the parking lot and sat in my car. Quannapowitt was a quiet, peaceful lake, with park benches, swings, a softball field, and tall green trees swaying in the breeze. Moms with baby strollers, men walking dogs, runners, and casual walkers made their way around the water. I admired the beauty all around me, and I prayed.

I opened my Bible and read. I'm not sure what I read, I just read and read. I was still thinking about our meeting with the doctors, but as I read, my anxiety started to diminish. As I read and prayed, I felt more confident that what I felt was right. It wasn't my mind playing tricks on me, and it wasn't me being delusional or stubborn. It was me being led, led by God. But I know God was speaking "truth" to me. Maybe that truth was just for me, to have as my safety net, my life preserver. I didn't try to articulate it, just trust and let the events unfold, a very difficult task but…

But again I had no choice, and I liked the peace and comfort I felt when I read my Bible and prayed. I sat for a few moments longer, enjoying the peaceful feeling. I took a deep breath, started my car, and headed home. I knew I had a battle on my hands, and nothing had changed, but I felt more confident and prepared than when I had left the hospital earlier.

As I walked in the door, my mother and Michael were happy to see me. My mom had prepared a dinner of pasta and meatballs, a favorite of the whole family. I sat with my mom and explained what the doctors had to say in our meeting.

"I just feel that everything will be all right," I told her.

Great mom that she is, she hugged me and said, "I have the utmost confidence in you, and if you feel that Michael will be fine, then I do too!" My mom was great that way; she always had my back. She headed back home to Winthrop.

When Mark came home, we enjoyed a normal dinner, as if nothing was wrong. But afterward, I just couldn't hold it in any longer. "Michael will be all right, he will survive," I said.

"You don't get it!" Mark replied. "Didn't you hear the doctors? Didn't you see the MRI?"

"I can't explain it. It's just something I feel." And as the words came out of my mouth, I realized how crazy I must have sounded. I'd seen everything he'd seen, heard what he'd heard, but I knew God was speaking to me and me alone.

"You'd better start praying that Michael survives the radiation."

And again I realized that my faith was simply that: mine. Mark wasn't there, and I couldn't get him there. I realized that he needed to find it on his own. Once I knew he would get there on his own, I stopped getting mad at his remarks. I'm sure he was trying to sort this all out in his mind, deal with his anger and sadness and at the same time thinking, *What is happening to my wife? Is she losing it?*

I wasn't arguing that the doctors were wrong; I was arguing how I felt, and I felt that Michael would be fine.

Dr. Ebb called a few days later to schedule another test for Michael, an experimental chemotherapy study which involved the chemo being injected into Michael's spinal fluid twice a week for three weeks. Dr. Ebb was skeptical; we needed to see if the spinal fluid at the base of his spine communicated thoroughly to his brain, with no blockages. But at least it was an option, and for the moment I didn't have to think about Michael having radiation. The test was mandatory if Michael was to participate in the study. I was uncertain about the whole thing but allowed the tests.

Once again, Michael and I were off to MGH to be poked and pinched. It was very hard to make a seven-year-old curl up in the fetal position while a nurse injects a needle into his spine. It didn't go well, and the nurse had to get help to hold Michael in the correct position. A mother's nightmare—people holding your son down as others poked him with needles. In the end, we were unsuccessful that day and would have to attempt it the next day, with the help of anesthesia.

We were back at MGH at 7:00 a.m. the next day. That's when we met one of the most amazing nurses.

Mary Rae was one of those people who could light up a room. She was in her late thirties with short, blond, curly hair. Average height, medium build, and everyday looking; she didn't wear makeup or anything flashy. And she was easygoing, optimistic, friendly, and compassionate. Even though it was her day off, Mary Rae had heard what Michael needed and offered to come in and help get it done.

I was mad to have to be there at all, after having been there just hours earlier watching the torture of my son. Mary Rae calmed me with her words and demeanor. She made Michael and me laugh and made the day a relatively fun experience.

My sister Anne is a nurse, and I know what an incredible person she is. I saw it in Mary Rae that day.

Dr. Ebb called later in the evening. "The testing went well," he said. "Michael can start the experimental drug the next week."

But I sensed that something wasn't right. "Will there be any more MRIs before the new drug therapy starts?"

"Yes, an MRI is needed within two weeks of starting the new therapy, as part of the drug protocol."

"That's it," I said. "That's it, there will be something different, something new." I just knew it.

Dr. Ebb was probably shocked at my response, but I didn't feel the need to explain. I had my own reasons for being happy, and promised to have Michael at MGH on Friday for his MRI. I hung up the phone, jumped for joy, and thanked God. My insides were screaming, "*Yes*," and my heart swelled.

Even though it may not have made sense "logically," I felt in my heart that the MRI would show good news. I had prayed about Michael being healed and felt so positive that it was possible. The feeling stayed with me; through the meetings with Ebb and Tarbell, through the spinal test, through talking with Ebb on the phone. I felt that a spirit was speaking to me, not my head.

On Friday, we made our journey once more to MGH, Mark, Michael, and me. Again we played the waiting game while Michael was in the MRI machine. We wrapped ourselves in warm blankets in the recovery room and sat and waited. Michael finally woke up, and we were on our way home. We made one stop: the Pancake House. It didn't matter what time it was, Michael always wanted breakfast—pancakes, eggs over medium, and bacon. So we stopped and ate, and once again I enjoyed the experience of eating with Mark and Michael, and seeing Michael dig into real food.

Later that night, Mark, Michael, and I watched TV waiting for the phone to ring. I pretended to watch with them but had no idea what was on. I couldn't focus; I just wanted to know! I stared at the phone and prayed for it to ring. Finally, around seven, the phone rang. It was Dr. Ebb.

"There's a change: the MRI shows no signs of tumor growth. In fact, it looks better than the original MRI."

I was stunned but happy. "Why the change?"

"It seems the MRI that showed that cancer growth was read incorrectly by the radiologist. Since Michael has contrast, the MRIs must always be read in the same order, from the head down. The incorrect MRI had been read from spine up. In doing so, the dye looked darker, appearing as if the cancer was growing compared to the previous MRI."

"Wow."

"In the future, I will only allow the chief radiologist read and report on Michael's MRIs. Since they're over one hundred pictures and very complicated, it would be best if the chief read them and myself, who are most familiar with Michael's complicated history."

"Thank you, Dr. Ebb. Thank you for the good news." I hung the phone and grinned at Mark and Michael. The end result? No radiation, no experimental drugs injected into Michael's spine. We were back to basics, back to our familiar protocol of chemotherapy and Irinotecan.

From the day we found out that his cancer was growing to the day we found it out was about six weeks. I felt like I was in the middle of a raging storm with an unbelievable center eye of inner peace. I can't explain it any better than that. I just think of Mary Stevenson's poem: "Footprints in the Sand." (http://www.footprints-inthe-sand.com/)

Footprints in the Sand

One night I dreamed I was walking along
the beach with the Lord.
Many scenes from my life flashed across the sky.
In each scene I noticed footprints in the sand.
Sometimes there were two sets of footprints,
other times there were one set of footprints.

This bothered me because I noticed
that during the low periods of my life,
when I was suffering from
anguish, sorrow or defeat,
I could see only one set of footprints.

So I said to the Lord,
"You promised me Lord,
that if I followed you,
you would walk with me always.
But I have noticed that during
the most trying periods of my life
there have only been one
set of footprints in the sand.
Why, when I needed you most,
you have not been there for me?"

The Lord replied,
"The times when you have
seen only one set of footprints in the sand,
is when I carried you."

For those six weeks, Jesus definitely carried me because there is no explanation for how I felt. And I was the only one feeling this way. I tried to explain it to others but quickly realized that wasn't what I was supposed to do. I was just supposed to believe, have faith and trust, to leave everything else up to God. He changes hearts, not me.

As busy as a normal family is, we were even busier with Michael's treatments. I constantly struggled to find time for "me." Family, laundry, grocery shopping, cooking, cleaning, and all of the other tasks of being a mom were taking a toll. Michael was still having his weekly chemo and occasional hospital visits. I think that's what started the early morning workouts at the gym at 5:30 a.m. so that I could be home by 7:00 to get the kids up, fed, and off to school. By 9:00 p.m., I was done, physically and mentally, day in and day out. Still, it was all part of the plan.

Some days I felt like I wasn't part of the real world. Before Michael was diagnosed, the real world meant work, gym, care of kids, chauffeuring, cooking, cleaning, socializing, vacation planning—basically, doing what one wanted. Once Michael was diagnosed, the days took on a different meaning, not what one wished to do but what needed to be done: hospitals, nurses, medications, doctors, phone calls, PT, and OT. No planning for vacations. Everything that took place in our lives had to be sanctioned by doctors. Going on a trip needed an okay from Michael's doctors. If Michael had any fluid in his head, he could not travel in a plane due to cabin pressure. Also, his chemo schedule dictated whether we would vacation. He had six weeks on, two weeks off chemotherapy, so we could only travel during those two weeks. Add to the mix two other children who could only travel during school vacations so they wouldn't miss a lot of work *and* your husband's work schedule, and it was next to impossible to make it all work out.

I did enjoy my days home with Michael that year. We watched *Teletubbies* a lot. No expectations, just taking care of him. Pauline or Arlyne would stop by with food or an offer to do laundry. I usually didn't leave the house except to take Michael swimming or to the hospital, until one day my friend Jean called.

"Hey, I'm taking tennis lessons around the corner at Northeast Tennis, and my partner can't make it this afternoon. Would you be interested in playing, just this one time?"

I'd first met Jean in 1983 when she was dating Mark's best friend, Joe. We often found ourselves on double dates, so we really had a chance to get to know each other. Jean was about five-eight, lean, fit, and attractive. She had curly brown hair, brown eyes, and an easy, fun personality. She lived around the corner, and we'd kept in touch all these years.

"Come on, Jodi. Just this time."

I thought for a moment and realized that it may not be a bad idea. It was only for an hour, and just around the corner. If my mom needed me, I could be home in minutes. I decided to give it a try. "Sure, let's do it," I said.

Jean picked me up, with me nervous to leave Michael but excited to be part of the real world. I felt like Jodi again. We played, and I had a blast. When I got home, Michael was fine. After five years of dealing with Michael's cancer and the restrictions on my schedule, my first trip out alone felt good. I had missed allowing me to be *me*. On occasion, I would join Jean for that tennis lesson and truly enjoy it.

Of course, as a friend who knew me pretty well, Jean knew that once I had a tennis racket in my hand, I would enjoy it so much that she wouldn't have to twist my arm to join her again. Also, she kept the "no commitment" plan. "I'll just call you when we need a fourth."

She did that with the gym too. "Got a week's free pass to the gym," she would say. "Just try it, no commitment—it's free." So again I'd try it, and Jean knew that once I started to lift weights—which I loved—and run and spin, it would be all over. No convincing or arm-twisting necessary. I enjoyed that week at the gym and knew that someday when Michael was better and attending a full day of school that the gym could become part of my life again.

Having a friend like Jean at a time like this was a blessing to me. She knew what I needed most of the time before I did. She never pressured me into anything but was always there to support me and my family. She drove Kaitlin back and forth to preschool for me, all with a smile on her face. She played songs in her car for Kaitlin like "Jungle Love" and the theme from "Golden Girls" as they went off to school. Kaitlin would then sing these songs at home; I often wondered where Kaitlin got those songs. It wasn't until years later I realized it was Jean!

Many days I longed for my old life back, before Michael was diagnosed, but I knew I was a better person, friend, sister, wife, and daughter than I was before. The pain and fear of what we went through hurt so much. I wouldn't want that for anyone. I do feel that it has made my children, Mark, and me stronger and more understanding of others.

Little did I know that yet another challenge was approaching, one that blindsided all of us.

CHAPTER 13

The Stars Have It

IT WAS A TYPICAL SEPTEMBER morning in 2006, and I was taking a much-needed shower after one of my morning spin classes when I noticed a lump in my right breast. I asked Mark to feel it, and he said, "Yup, it's a lump," and that he had never felt it before. I was scheduled for a routine mammogram at the end of the month so didn't think about the lump again until my appointment.

Once there, I had my gown down to my waist and those awkward half-naked moments going on. "I have felt a lump in my right breast," I said.

"Oh, then I'll have the radiologist look at the films right away since you've got a concern." She came after a few minutes and said, "The right breast showed no abnormalities, but you do have dense breasts. If you want, you can have an ultrasound."

I almost said no; after all, I had a million things to do. "Okay, then, let's go ahead." I lay out on the stretcher and the tech squeezed that cold goop onto my breasts, then pressed the cold wand onto them.

"Yes," she said. "Dense right breast." So it was unanimous that I have a dense right breast. I could live with that. I wiped off the goop with the harsh paper towels, feeling relieved. Off I went from the hospital to go about my day.

About a week later, an older woman at my church died of breast cancer. I had served with her on several committees and had enjoyed her devotion and dedication to our parish. I decided to attend the funeral. As I walked into the church, a greeter attached a pink ribbon to the right lapel of my jacket. The mass was beautiful and tearful. I went home and, as usual, didn't' even have a chance to get my coat off before I was called to one chore or another. I was making Jordan's bed when the phone rang.

It was the doctor's office. "Your mammogram revealed 'suspicious spots' in my left breast, and we want to do a biopsy."

"But the lump was in my right breast," I reminded her. "The technician had determined the cause to be dense breast tissue."

She said, "It's not your right breast but your left."

My left breast? I hadn't felt anything on my left breast. What was going on?

"Maybe you have the wrong person," I tried. "My real name is Josephine, and I go by Jodi. Can you please check for me?" She put me on hold, and I listened to that awful elevator music.

"No, this information is correct. You need a biopsy."

I continued to argue with her. She was very polite and never seemed to get aggravated with me. I finally conceded and took down the name and number of the doctor they wanted to contact for the biopsy.

I hung up the phone and sat on the end of Jordan's bed, stroking the pink ribbon on my right lapel. As much as I wanted to believe this was not happening, I also knew in my heart and soul what was going on. I have had this same feeling before when Michael was first sick, and no one could figure out the case. It was knowing the truth, yet at the same time trying so hard to convince my mind that I wasn't crazy and what I was feeling was not the truth. But I knew, "the Big C" had invaded my home once again!

I ran downstairs to tell Mark. He comforted me with, "Don't worry, it may be nothing." He's the kind of guy who only worries when he has to. Until he knows and has answers, no worries!

"Maybe so," I agreed with him, but as much as I tried to convince my mind, my heart and soul were conflicted.

I called Dr. Ebb, whom I had come to trust, and told him what was going on. I asked him, "If it was your wife, who would you send her to?"

"Dr. Barbra Smith," he answered.

Dr. Ebb was kind enough to get me a difficult appointment. If I had cancer, then I am going to MGH. If they could help Michael with life-threatening cancer, they could certainly help me. I gathered referrals, mammograms, and ultrasound reports, and off to MGH Mark and I went, thankfully without Michael this time.

Once at the radiologist's clinic, I was told to use locker number ten. "Hold onto your purse, there are no locks. Take off everything from the waist up"—typical marching orders for all women about to have a mammogram. MGH preferred that their own technicians take images for diagnostic purposes, so I was waiting for my turn in a cold waiting room.

Partly because I worked as a technical clothing designer, I always noticed patient garb, whether it was for Michael or me. The gowns provided for mammograms are "one size fits all," and could cover my body and that of four friends. They opened in the front, which provided little security for the modest. There was exposed flesh all over the waiting room.

Mammograms had always been a no-brainer, as they are for many women, but now I'd come with a little more anxiety in my heart. I know in the end that everything would be okay, it was the journey to the end that made me nervous. What if they confirmed the suspicious thing was cancer? How would I react? I just sat and stared at the ugly green walls.

They called my name, and off I went to the most uncomfortable test imaginable, and I thought: *If I had bigger breasts, this damned test would not hurt so much.* They tried to put my small breast in a vice grip and get my body out of the way at the same time, a physiological challenge.

Twenty minutes later, the mammogram was done, and Mark and I were once again walking the halls of MGH. Same familiar building, Yawkey, same pale hallways. We boarded the elevator and I pushed the button for the eighth floor. As we stood silently in the elevator, I realized I pushed the wrong button. I was so used to going to the eighth floor to see Dr. Ebb that I just did it automatically. What was wrong with my brain? It hadn't caught up with what was actually happening!

I pushed another button for the ninth floor to meet my new surgeon, Dr. Barbara Smith. We signed in and produced all the necessary information identification: driver's license, health insurance card, and the most holy-of-holy cards, the "MGH Blue Card." It had a patient reference number that allowed the hospital to access all of your medical info, along with billing and health insurance. Never leave home without it. You couldn't get anywhere in MGH without this card.

I often thought that MGH should have different-colored cards. Like the airlines, gold or platinum, depending on your frequency. Yes, I felt I should have some special privileges since I was there weekly. A parking discount, perhaps, or a free snack, no-wait check-in, maybe? That would be nice. I would most certainly be a platinum member! Not something I would brag about, but it would sure help ease the pain of all the expenses and inconvenience we have had to endure during our considerable time in this hospital.

"No frequent flyer discount?" I asked the girl checking me in. She just smiled and asked for me driver's license. I ask, "Why do you need to see my driver's license?"

"To see a picture ID to make sure you are who you say you are."

Really? How many women willingly walk in to an oncologist's office pretending to be someone else? Honestly, I didn't want to be there, and I couldn't imagine someone pretending to be me.

Once called, we entered a small examining room. I got weighed and asked to take everything off from the waist up. I'd heard those words way too many times lately. Again I don the adorable robe, open in the front, and tie it, an act of futility.

Dr. Smith knocked at the door and in walks a beautiful tall blonde woman with short, sassy hair, wearing a well-fitting Ann Taylor–like navy suit. This woman could be a model! And I thought, *She could be my friend.* Her demeanor was warm and reassuring.

She did a breast exam.

"What about the lump on my right breast?" I asked. Couldn't seem to leave that alone.

"I'm not too concerned about it. It's most likely nothing, just part of your breasts being dense." She was calm and controlled, and didn't seem alarmed about the lump.

"If you had a lump in your breast that everyone said was fine, what would you do?"

She immediately says, "I would remove it." That was when I relaxed and immediately liked her even more. I got dressed, and Mark and I met Dr. Smith in her office to review the most recent mammogram.

"I agree that the suspicious shadows on your left breast are clusters of small dots that light up greyish."

I knew what to look for, as I have read many similar scans. You never want to see any greyish areas on scans. That much I knew. We looked again at the lump on my right breast, still convinced it was nothing but agreed it should be removed. We scheduled a biopsy for both breasts on Monday, but I wouldn't have the results until the end of the week. What a long week it will be.

I knew what to do, I had been there before with Michael. I prayed, read, and asked God for help and healing. I had a week to prepare myself, and I did just that. I kept to my exercise routine, ate healthy food, and prayed. I needed to be ready physically, mentally, and spiritually for Monday. I knew that would bolster my chances of success, of peace.

Monday morning came, and Mark and I made the trek back to MGH for a procedure to pinpoint exactly the spot the biopsy should target. This was done on my left beast only. There were clusters of small dots, and they needed to make sure they got the problematic cluster.

The procedure involved squishing my breast into a mammogram-like device, after which the technician inserts very fine wires through your breast and out the other side. The technician monitored this all on a screen which, hopefully, clearly shows the markings of the area to be biopsied. She then tried to capture that same area on your breast and insert the wires. There was a strong sting and slight pain and then nothing. The wire was through one side of your breast and hung out your other side.

Because I had such small, dense breasts, this was not easy, simple, or quick. The tech determined she'd gotten the wrong spot, and we start again. They freed my poor breast for a breather.

There were two people in the room with me, the technician and a nurse. They asked now and then, "Are you all right?" I just answered yes. What do you say, no? That wouldn't get me out of this mess. But both were very nice and comforting. The nurse rubbed my back as the technician again and again inserted the wires. By now I am sweating profusely, saying Hail Mary's, and Our Father's. Thank God for those rote prayers I had memorized as a child.

Finally we were done, and I was wheeled into the waiting room with my "one size fits nobody" robe and five wires protruding through my breast! I climbed onto the cold, hard stiff sheets of the gurney in prep for the operating room. Now I knew, truly, how Michael feels: uneasy, scared, nervous.

The nurses got my IV running, and Mark and I visited with the anesthesiologist. Many of the nurses recognized me but were not sure because I was always with Michael. They cocked their heads and said, "Jodi? What's going on?" They're not used to seeing *me* on the gurney.

All were very comforting and caring. What great nurses I have met with all my visits to MGH. I am ready for my "cocktail," as the anesthesiologist put it, just something to relax me.

"You'll just feel like you've had a glass of wine or two." Okay, that's good, a little something to take the edge off! I kissed Mark good-bye, and off he went, to patiently wait. We've gotten so good at that.

I was ready, and so were the surgeons and the team that will be with me in the operating room. I was wheeled into a very bright, cold, and shiny operating room. As they transferred me from the gurney onto the operating table, my gown (already becoming a problem) loosened and opened up, exposing more flesh than I would prefer. No one seemed to notice, and the team continued to prep for surgery. My arms were held down with Velcro. I couldn't move now, nor did I care that my one size fits nobody gown was hanging off of me! I am peaceful and relaxed.

"Hi," Dr. Smith said as she leaned over me. She discreetly covered me up. Thank God for women taking care of women.

The next thing I knew, the mask was on my face. "Count down from ten." I didn't make it past eight.

I woke up with ice packs on my chest and very groggy. Dr. Smith had already reported to Mark, who was patiently waiting, that everything looked good. The lump on the right was taken out and sent off to pathology, but it looked pretty good to her. Same with the cluster on the left breast. When I'm released, Mark and I head home for the waiting game. It was Monday, and I won't know anything until the end of the week.

When I got home, I just went to bed. Mark often worked from home, so was able to help take care of me. By Wednesday, I was feeling more like myself, but still no news. I called Dr. Smith Wednesday afternoon, but results had not come in.

By Friday, I still had heard nothing. I was having Father Mike, my parish priest, over for dinner, so I was preoccupied with planning dinner and distracted with the kids. The phone rang at 6:00 p.m. The caller ID told me it was Dr. Smith. I sat down at the kitchen table.

She said very calmly, "The left breast that showed suspicious shadowing is fine."

What a relief! The right breast with the lump is probably fine too, is what I think. All the doctors agreed that dense breasts make concrete diagnoses difficult.

But then I heard it, "However, the right breast that had the lump is cancer. I'm sorry to have to give you this news. Please call my office on Monday, and we'll schedule another biopsy on the right breast. I need to go back in and take additional tissue. The margins weren't clean enough the first time."

I hung up the phone and started to cry. Mark came in from the living room and just held me. "The right breast has cancer," I sobbed. "Cancer again!"

We didn't say much for a while, just stood together and hugged. Mark was always very cautious and calm about things. "Let's not get too worked up yet. Let's get the other biopsy done. It's not life-threatening, and we can get it all fixed."

But I felt like, *Here we go again. The "Big C" is back to rule my life!*

Deep down, I was hoping the doctor was wrong. I'd always said, "Just because you have an MD next to your name, that doesn't mean you are always right!" I had so many instances with Michael's care over the years when doctors would say things like, "He won't live six months," or "He won't live to be three years old…four years old," or "His eyesight won't come back," or "His hearing will be compromised." And none of it came true.

I just listened and believe what I believe: doctors are not always right. I put my faith in God. He was always in control, even though things sometimes seem hopeless. There was always a better plan.

That Friday night, Mark and I decided to keep the news to ourselves for a while. The doorbell rang, and Father Mike came in for dinner. I so wanted to say something, but just couldn't. I was still in shock.

But later that weekend, we told the kids and assured them it was nothing like Michael's cancer, telling them that Michael's cancer was life-threatening, but mine was treatable. I could tell by the look on their faces that they were scared. It had been eight years since Michael's diagnosis in '98, but the turmoil and the grief they experienced was still very much on their minds. I felt like my children were growing up so fast, having to deal with so many adult issues at such a young age. On some level though, all this heartache prompted such great conversations about life faith.

The conversations I had with Michael were very different. One afternoon the next week, I was walked home from the bus stop with him. "Michael, I need to tell you something important. I'm going to have an MRI and surgery later on this week."

He stopped, turned to me, and said, "Be brave, be brave, Mom." Simple, powerful words from a ten-year-old boy. At ten, Michael already knew too well what those words meant. I think that he had lived with this phrase for a very long time, these simple yet challenging words.

We hugged and walked home. Sometimes I thought, *Wow! My kids are dealing with such heavy stuff. Are they getting cheated out of their innocent lives as children?* But I can't change our lives, and continue to see the good in having all these talks with them. I also feel that my children have learned so much through our family's many experiences. They seem more accepting of others, more tolerant, compassionate. I could see it already—light coming out of the dark.

The following weeks were all about scheduling surgery. Dr. Smith performed a second biopsy but still didn't get clean margins, so a third biopsy was performed. With that, we finally had clean margins, and no more surgeries. After all those biopsies though, my right breast was left with divots, kind of like a shooting gallery. My breast tissue was pretty much gone, and I was left with a boob that looked like an egg over-easy—flat and round! No real complaints, I could have been left with no breast at all. I've learned to always look for optimistic alternatives. This helped me come to grips with what could have been. I came out of all this pretty lucky, and was grateful for my minor surgeries. I don't have to look too far to see what could have been!

I had a month free of the hospital, and then had to start radiation. My protocol was eight weeks of radiation every weekday. So at 7:20 a.m. each morning, I would be at MGH—my second home once again!

I remember pulling up to the hospital valet the first day of radiation and seeing a warm, familiar face—"Mac," a tall, handsome black man whose accent when greeting me always belied his island background. Mac always parked my car when I came to the hospital with Michael. He gave me a big hug, asked about Michael, and took my car safely away.

My "second home" had an eerily welcoming feeling. I went downstairs to check in and donned the one size fits no one gown.

Can't we sit here in something a little more fashionable—better fabric, more cheerful colors, a more flattering shape? Could we try to distinguish men's gowns from women's? Can we just borrow the same gown for eight weeks at a time then burn it, instead of wearing the gown for twenty minutes, then throwing it in the laundry?

As I tried to design a new gown in my head, I saw another familiar face coming toward me—Sheila Brown, Michael's nurse who had switched from pediatric oncology to adult oncology. We talked, hugged, cried, and had a few laughs about the days past. I pulled out pictures of Michael and brought Sheila up to speed on his progress.

I never thought I would be at the MGH adult cancer center. Somehow I just thought that I was done with the cancer thing and that someone else would now get a turn with it. Honestly, I was mad. Someone else should have been stuck with this. If your son had been diagnosed with a brain tumor and given six months to live, shouldn't that exempt other family members from the nightmare? I know now that it's not how it works, but in my current frame of mind, I was counting on that theory. Once I realized that the theory doesn't work, and I indeed had cancer, the challenge was on.

I hear my name, "Josephine," and carefully hold my gown closed as I walk to my nurse, a young girl with a cheery smile. She was soft-spoken and cute, and very pregnant. I lied on a cold metal stretcher and took my arm out of my right sleeve, exposing my breast. They lined up a giant machine over my right breast, so close to my body I had to close my eyes to fight claustrophobia.

The week prior, they had given me four "tattoos," that gave them a map for positioning the machine for radiation. Each time I come, they would know exactly where to place the machine to radiate only the designated area.

"If I'm getting the tattoo, can I have a star?" I'd asked jokingly.

"No," the technician said, "only blue dots."

Those people should really lighten up. Another great idea down the drain!

The pregnant nurse asked me what I want to listen to. "A little *Boston* would be good," I said.

"Peace of Mind" came through the headphones and we were ready to roll. The nurse left the room, and I was alone with the music. The machine started up and began to move very slowly, closely over my right breast. I closed my eyes and concentrated on the music. Within minutes, the pregnant girl was back.

"All done, see you tomorrow."

And I was off to start my day.

For nine months, I'd been going to the gym and had even hired a personal trainer, Peter Reppas. I'd seen him working with another woman about my age, using Velcro bands and doing leg lifts, and it looked both challenging and effective. I initially planned for ten visits to get me on track with weight lifting and to help me get a handle on my "thunder thighs." At five feet, three inches tall and one hundred-thirty pounds, my short legs held a good portion of my weight. With a petite waist and upper body though, I hid my weight well; no one would ever guess I weighted that much.

But after my ten visits with Peter, I was so happy with the results that I signed on for ten more, then ten more and ten more. Two and a half years later, Peter still motivated me, inspiring me to do more. Once I accomplish a goal I set out to do, Peter always asked, "So what's next?" or "You need to step it up." I loved it.

I can still remember telling Peter I had cancer. I was in the corner of the gym on the lat pull-down machine. Peter knew I was having surgeries as I had to cut back on my training schedule. He came up to me and said, "What's the word?"

"I have cancer." That's all I said. I didn't look up but continued to pull down with all my strength on the handles. I finally had to stop and look at him.

"The man from above has given you a test, and you will pass," he said. "You are ready. You can handle this."

Really? I thought. Not me. I was done, I felt defeated.

The afternoon, after my visit to MGH for my first radiation treatment, I received an e-mail from Peter. It went like this:

> > From: Peter Reppas
> > Subject: Jodi's 7 Week Plan
> > To: "Jodi Sampson"
> > Date: Friday, February 2, 2007, 2:02 PM Hi,
> >
> *Okay here we go! Starting the week after next, you will pick the four days during the week Monday thru Friday, that work best for you to meet @ 10am. The goal will be to get the four days in during the week, because if a glitch*

*happens, you will have Saturday and Sunday to make up
for it if necessary.*

*Each week will count as a session! I don't have to do
this, I want to do this and I think it is very important for
your 'funkiness' to stay on point as much as possible during
those 7 weeks. Because, realistically, those are some of the
most important weeks of your life if you think about it. You
are trying to get rid of something that is life-threatening
and you have a family that relies on you dearly.*

*So the goal is to KEEP you the strongest physically,
mentally and spiritually that you have ever been during
this time. I don't have to worry about you spiritually!
Physically and mentally we can get out of rhythm and
that is not allowed! Ill do my part if you do yours.*

Good! Now I feel better! Enjoy your day!

I guess it should never have come to a surprise to me that
Peter would step up to the plate and be there as a great friend
for support. I remember being in the gym on one particular
Sunday, and I never went to the gym on Sundays. I was on
the elliptical machine.

Peter walked up. "What are you doing here?"

"Too cold to run outside, so I came indoors," I replied.

"I just got back from church, where I lit a candle and
prayed for you."

I thought I would fall off the machine. I was speechless.
No words, just gratitude and an aha moment. God truly puts
people in our path for a reason. Throughout my life, many

have said they prayed for Michael, but never just for me. I was blessed to have a friend who understood the importance of prayer and what it means to me!

That afternoon, reading his e-mail, I felt so much better. He had such confidence in me. Why wasn't I that confident in myself? Would he do his part if I do mine? *Wow!* How could I lose? I knew right then and there that I was going to be fine through all of this and yes, God has prepared me for this journey. I would survive, with all the family and friends who surround me today!

This is going to be the best eight weeks of your life!" Peter told me.

"You're f—— nuts!" I snapped back, but he made it come true.

I saw Peter three days a week during my radiation treatment. I met him after radiation and before work. Having to meet someone at the gym who gave up his time freely committed to help me succeed—how could I not go? He always greeted me with a smile, saying, "Tell me something good, boss!"

One day, as I opened my weight lifting notebook to start my workout with Peter, all these star stickers fell out. Peter had made up a calendar, starting with my first day of radiation to my last day. Each star represented an accomplishment on my part. (As it happens, the first treatment started on Ash Wednesday and ended on Good Friday. I had my own personal Lenten sacrifice that year.) It was fun to apply the stars after my workouts each day. Friday's gold star was my favorite. I always got five stars on Fridays. I had always used stickers and charts to motivate my kids, but I was very surprised that, at forty-five, stars still motivated me. Silly as it was, it got me through.

Stars carried a special meaning to me. They represented one of my favorite Bible stories. When Abraham was trying to have a child at a very old age, the Lord told him that he and Sara indeed would have a child. This was very hard for Sara and Abraham to believe, so the Lord took Abraham outside and had him look up to the stars. He said, "Abraham, your descendants will be as many as the stars."

Those gold stars were a constant reminder to me of all God's promises to all believers. Many times, when I ran early in the morning, it was still dark. Afterward, I would stand and stare up at the sky and the many stars and remember all of God's promises for me. Those stars are what kept me focused, faithful, and hopeful.

Our bodies are gifts, and the last time I checked, we only get one. After Michael and I were both diagnosed with cancer, I began to think about my body, as well as my family's bodies, as a temple. Before I was diagnosed, I had never thought too much about food as fuel. Once I started a serious exercise routine though, I needed all the right food to help me make it through the day. I saw such great results: less fatigue and lethargy, less moodiness. The better I felt, the more I wanted to live healthy, and to share it with my family. I also started appreciating my body for what it is, not what it's not. Hopefully, I've passed this on to my loved ones as well.

I've read many health, nutrition, fitness, and fashion magazines over the years, and realized how many women hate their bodies. I know many women who say that they can't look at themselves naked. One poll I read stated that 75 percent of women are not happy in the bodies in which they live, and plastic surgery is on the rise. Something is seriously wrong with the way women view their bodies. How sad to walk the earth with that self-image.

When did our bodies become something we hated, or didn't want to look at? When did our bodies become something that had to be perfect by someone else's standards? When did we start to think that to have a beautiful body meant plastic surgery to fix all the things that society and magazines say are wrong? I am not against plastic surgery. I just think we need to know where our happiness lies. Plastic surgery is a viable option for many, but happiness will not lie in perky breasts or a flat tummy. It needs to come from within.

Over the years, I'd learned and lamented about my body. I first began working out to lose weight and get rid of my "thunder thighs." I've changed my opinion on what our bodies are and what they should look like. I believe our bodies are more about who we are than what we think. If we are happy with our bodies, this happiness translates into our everyday lives. It reflects how we carry ourselves, our attitudes, and our self-image. I have always had a love/hate relationship with my body—love my abs, hate my thighs, want longer legs, need to lose ten pounds, want my perky boobs back, and love my arms. It wasn't until I was stricken with breast cancer, when my breasts got dissected and scarred with radiation, that I realized how much I totally love my body, not in an arrogant way, but in a peaceful and contented way.

On day, as I was changing, I ran into the laundry room off my bedroom. I had just returned from the gym and was removing my clothes and preparing a load of laundry, multitasking again. As I stripped down to my naked body, I passed my full-length mirror. Normally I would have kept on running and jumped into the shower, but today proved different. I stopped and looked at my naked body from all angles—front, side, and back. I looked at all of the scars.

The three-inch scar with the divot on my lower right side of my stomach from when I was seventeen and my appendix burst. The three scars in the center of my lower stomach from three C-sections. The small scar underneath my belly button from a laparoscopy after two miscarriages. The four small little blue tattoos from the radiation that surround my right breast. The scars on my right and left breasts from the surgery to remove cancer. The radiation burns that seem to encapsulate my right breast. The scars from reconstructive surgery. The difference between my right breast that sat about one inch higher than my left breast. I just stood there and looked.

I thought about what beauty really means. It's not the women on magazine covers that have been touched up for our viewing pleasure. It's about having the eyes to see beauty. I saw the beauty in my scarred and battled body. I did not see those scars as a liability, but as an asset. Those scars made me, *me*. Some have faded, but the memories of them are always with me.

For the first time in a long time, I realized such amazing beauty, inside and out. Finally I was proud to be Jodi Sampson, age forty-seven. Our bodies are a gift and say so much about who we are. I believe God gave me this body to learn, grow, and develop into the woman I saw in the mirror that day. I know God sees all my scars, inside and out, and says, *What beauty*. It is our job on this earth to have the eyes to see that beauty too. For if we see that beauty in ourselves, we can't help but see it in others. The beauty we feel will emanate in our lives and in the lives of others.

In the end, my cancer ordeal lasted from September through April. I had several resectioning surgeries and radiation treatment for eight weeks, five days a week. My cancer was treatable, and in April of 2007, I was considered fine. Though doctors will never use the term "cured" when it comes to cancer, I considered myself cured. With God's help and my faith, our family continued on with our "normal" life.

Jodi Journal Entry

I have learned to live in the moment, not in my past or think about my future. I pay attention to the present always. If I can concentrate on the present only I will find my happiness.

Since God can only live in the present with us, that is where I always want to be in the right now!

As I write my journal entry, I stop and think...there is so much life in this world and the stars in heaven constantly remind me.

Life can be fun, a party, a joy, because life is a collection of days, the moment we are living right now.

> *All who call upon Me, I will answer, I will be with them in distress; I will deliver them and give them honor. With length of days I will satisfy them and show them my saving power.*

—Psalm 91: 15, 16

CHAPTER 14

Life Goes On

AT 7:15 A.M., ON AN October day in 2007, I walked through the turnstile into MGH. I feel that I have just left. It amazed me how quickly I go back in my mind to the first day I walked into this place eight years ago. Feelings resurfaced automatically, the memories of feeling scared, and of the unknown. I had a love/hate relationship with this hospital. I hated being here: the smells, the sounds, the people, memories everywhere I look. Yet, I love it too. This hospital, the doctors, and all the people in here, saved Michael's life.

Michael was ten years old now, and his chemo treatment was done. He'd been on chemo steadily for about five years and so far, all MRIs indicated no tumor growth. The problem was that cancer cells looked the same in Michael's brain scans—the dead cells and the live ones. There was no way of knowing which were dead and which were still alive. Michael had extensive cancer throughout his head, and in layers of his brain, so a biopsy of every cell would be harmful and pointless because of the extensiveness of the disease.

Mark and I had talked with Dr. Ebb over time and at length about when to stop chemo. He assured us that if we stopped the chemo, one live cancer cell in Michael's brain could grow and multiply, eventually killing him. Honest, straightforward words from Dr. Ebb.

Mark and I discussed it, and prayed about it. By 2003 Michael was seven years old, and doing so great, we both felt confident that it was time to stop the chemo. We had peace about our decision and went ahead with it.

There were many other times in this journey with Michael that Mark and I had to make hard decisions and believe beyond what the doctors told us. One particular incident stands out in my mind. It was also in 2003. Shortly after Michael had his third shunt placed, his eyes crossed after surgery. The doctor explained it was temporary. Every morning, I got Michael out of his crib, not looking at him, walked downstairs with him in my arms, praying his eyes had reverted to normal, stood in the front hall, and then looked at him in the mirror. He was still cross-eyed. The girls said he had "googoo eyes."

Weeks went by, and Michael's right eye went back to normal, but his left eye was still crossed, so Dr. Butler, Michael's neurosurgeon, suggested we see a nuero ophthalmologist.

It was the Friday before the fourth of July, and the only appointment he had was 7:00 a.m. Mark, Michael, Kaitlin, and I made our way into Mass Eye and Ear to see the doctor, who performed several tests on Michael and determined that, because Michael's left eye had been crossed for a period of time, he had been seeing double. "The eye compensates by shutting the vision in that eye down," the doctor told us.

"What does that mean?" I asked.

"It means that Michael can't see out of his left eye."

"He's blind in one eye?"

"Yes."

And the next thing I knew it was 7:20, and I was saying good-bye to Mark who was heading off to work, both of us shocked and confused. My son had a brain tumor and is blind in one eye. How could I not see that? How could we not have known?

We went to Friendly's for breakfast, and I just sat there in disbelief. Michael and Kaitlin scarfed down eggs, pancakes, and bacon. I stared at Michael. He seemed fine to me. *That doctor is crazy!* I thought to myself.

About two weeks later, Michael's left eye started to go back to normal. We went out to Friday's for dinner, all five of us. I left the table to take Jordan to the ladies' room. While I was gone, Mark decided to play doctor.

When I got back to the table, Mark said, "Watch this." He placed a spoon over Michael's right eye. Mark help up a napkin and said, "What is this?"

"A napkin," Michael replied.

Mark held up a knife and said "What is this?"

"A knife," replied Michael. We went through everything on the table: salt, pepper, books, toys, menus, you name it. Michael saw everything clearly with his left eye! We all laughed so hard! Imagine, a simple spoon test at a casual family dinner determined that my son could see. I knew that doctor was crazy! I realized that evening at Friday's that Michael was no normal kid—no kid is—and sometimes general, stereotypical rules just don't apply.

Typical or not, today was a routine MRI, which Michael had once a year. I felt there wasn't much to worry about. Michael was doing well, and I suspected everything will be the same. He did require anesthesia because he had to remain still for two hours, a next-to-impossible task unless we drugged him. Michael remained cool and calm as we entered the clinic. All the nurses knew him and treated him like a celebrity. Debbie, Bob, and Mary Rae all greeted him and expressed their disbelief at how big he has gotten.

As I approached the MRI room, more memories flooded my mind—years of carrying Michael in and placing him onto this long stretcher. They wrapped him in warm blankets and gently placed his head in the narrow tube. Previous times, he'd barely covered a quarter of the stretcher. Today he walked into the MRI room and jumped onto the scanner, put his own head in the narrow tube, and covered himself with the warm blankets. His body was long and lean, and covered the entire stretcher. Bob, being the funny man he is, stayed with us, always cracking jokes and making Michael laugh.

They inserted the IV and slowly pumped Propofol into his veins, sedating him in preparation for the MRI. My left cheek rested on Michael's face as I held his hand. His eyes started to roll; he gave a big yawn and closed his eyes.

I kissed his lips and said, "I love you," and "Jesus is with you." I turned around, swallowed and took a deep breath as I left the cold room. Many thoughts crowded my mind: *I am blessed; I am grateful; I am appreciative; I am happy to be going home today.* On the other hand, I was hungry, and I didn't like being here. But how far we had come!

When I walked into MGH in 1998, I couldn't have known how big a part of my life this intuition would become. My first thought on that terrible day we got the news was that we'd be home by the weekend, having gotten answers and moved on. Then, when we got news of Michael's brain tumor I thought, *Okay, surgery, chemo six months to a year, we can do this!* Never did I think oncologists, surgeons, nurses, doctors, physiologists, and occupational and physical therapists, endocrinologist, neurosurgeons, and so many other doctors would be part of our life for so long. I've had the ability to have Michael treated by the best and most compassionate team of doctors. I have nothing but admiration for all of them.

Today, I felt the results of the MRI would be fine, no surprises. I always went by my heart and gut. I knew Michael and could always tell when something was wrong. I've never been surprised by what the doctors have told me, except for the initial diagnosis.

Outside, the leaves were turning beautiful colors—yellow, burnt orange, brick red, typical fall shades. The breeze was refreshing and blew my hair away from my face. I welcomed the coolness on my face after the hot summer days. Even though many people were all around me, I noticed only the scenery, gazing at the white fluffy clouds, and wishing I could jump on one and fly away. Their softness always look so inviting to me.

Mark and I went to the Jury Hotel, the old Charles Street jail, for breakfast in The Clink, a local and very cool restaurant. It had brick walls and black metal bars, very authentic.

"Coffee with milk please," I ordered. I stared out the window at a beautifully clear, crisp day, getting a little chilly.

Mark talked about Kaitlin and her soccer game the night before. "Her team is doing well," he said, "going to States."

I chatted and listened, but my mind was with Michael. Some things just don't get easier. I felt like I could cry, and I wanted to, but didn't. I don't really know why I felt that way. Everything was good, and Michael was healthy. Just my emotions. The leaves were turning, and it was a glorious day in Boston. I glanced out the window again and said, "Thank you, Jesus, for today."

Mark and I finished our breakfast and walked back to MGH. I reveled in the cool, brisk fall air and tried to enjoy the beauty that surrounded me for the moment.

We headed down the hallway toward the MRI room to see Michael. Waiting has become a real job. The medical community seemed to function at a different pace and operate by a different clock than the rest of us. Michael's scan should have taken two hours, but two hours had come and gone, and Michael was still in the scanner.

Around us, patients waiting their turn lay on stretchers, drinking the required white, milky substance through a straw. I couldn't help but think that no matter how healthy you may be, everyone looks sick lying on a stretcher in a hospital gown. I needed to design brighter, more colorful, fresher-looking gowns. Anything to make us feel better.

There were chairs for those of us who are the "waiters." I felt a little more at ease. Perhaps the hazelnut French toast, fruit, and coffee helped. Yeah, that was it—food always helps. At seventeen dollars though, I felt guilty eating only half. What a waste. Maybe it was my Catholic school upbringing that made me feel this way.

In Catholic school, Sister Adunata walked the cafeteria and made sure we all ate all of the lunches our mothers had packed for us, including the crust on the sandwiches! She was a little bit of a thing, only five feet tall in her full black habit. You could only see her hands and face. I always wondered if she had hair. She walked slowly and methodically up and down the cafeteria, saying with a deep stern voice, "Children are starving in Burma." I had no clue where Burma was, and I'm pretty sure most of the others kids didn't either. I was one of the members of the clean plate club, always ate my lunch, and never wanted to get on Sister Adunata's bad side.

Still waiting. Stretchers were wheeled by, doors opened and closed, but there was no sign of Michael yet. I knew he was fine; I just wanted to see him and hold his hand. I am a visual person; I love to see it! I tell myself to be patient, that before I know it we will be back in the car heading home to Middleton.

Eventually the doors swung open, and Michael was wheeled out complete with warm white blankets surrounding him. Deb, his nurse, was right beside him. Michael was wheeled into the waiting area, where we sat and waited for him to wake up. Mark and I sat beside his bed and gazed at him. Not sure what we were looking for, just looking. As we watched, Michael started to shake uncontrollably, and we called Deb back in. She had to call the anesthesiologist, and we waited some more.

Was he having a seizure? Was he cold? What is going on? I'd never seen this before. He just lay there, his body wrapped in blankets, eyes closed, body shaking. The anesthesiologist arrived and examined Michael.

"I think this is a reaction due to the anesthesia and the coldness of the MRI room. His body is adjusting to the different temperatures."

I am happy for this simple answer, but still didn't like to see Michael shake. It reminded me too much of the time he had a major seizure. I hugged him and tried to stop him from shaking. Eventually he stopped and we called his name, helping him wake up.

"Michael, Michael, wake up, baby. You're back with us. Wake up."

He finally opened one eye. Great, a sign we were on our way out the door! Michael eventually woke up completely, and we got him dressed and carefully take our "to go" bag, a brown paper bag with apple juice, saltines, and graham crackers. We said good-bye and headed for the door. We didn't wait around to get the results.

Michael's scans were very complicated, and they needed to be carefully compared to last year's scans. I know we'll get a call later from Dr. Ebb, so for now we are free. As Mark drove us home, I sat in the back seat with Michael, still a bit drowsy. I just liked to be next to him and hold his hand. He was getting hungry, so we stopped at the Pancake House for the usual—two eggs over medium, bacon and a pancake. He ate everything!

"My breath smells," he complained after finishing his food.

"It's from the anesthesia, hon," I explain. "It will wear off."

As Mark pressed the garage door opener at home, I realized that I was glad today was over. I knew that the journey with Michael would always be filled with ups and downs. Today we were on an up, and are grateful for it. I'd come to cherish the "good" days, as I knew tomorrow could and will be different. The simple things in life made me happy; I didn't get upset with the little things, and I didn't let people get to me. I kept myself centered in daily prayer to give me the strength to endure and "let it all go."

We were home and able to sleep in our own beds. Today was behind us, and I was very happy about that!

-»)«-

We'd long put off the kids about getting a dog. Of course, they'd always wanted a dog, but while we were navigating the medical world of Michael's illness…

"It's just too much for us," I tried to explain to the kids. "I have a hard enough time taking care of you and the house. And you know how many emergency visits and hospital stays we have to deal with."

Their faces fell, but I think they understood, disappointed as they might have been. But we did promise them that when Michael was cancer-free and we'd had a more normal life, we would get a dog.

We never discussed what breed; Mark had a golden retriever as a child, Gal, and loved her dearly. It seemed a great breed for us in every way, very family-friendly, and with such cute puppies, no one argued about getting another retriever.

So when Michael was off chemo and life resumed to "normal" in 2003, we got Boomer. The greatest decision ever. Boomer was a tangible sign to me of Michael's victory.

Even though life with the challenges of Michael's illness were arduous, he managed to have a pretty great life. At age eleven, he was in fifth grade, and he had many people in his life who helped him on a daily basis outside of school. Because of Michael's brain damage, he wasn't able to keep up with kids his own age physically and mentally, so even sports and any activity could be difficult.

Michael loved to swim, and so when we wanted Michael to continue with swimming lessons without me in the pool, it was a challenge. I was such a big part of Michael's life, but I needed others to do the things that I wasn't good at or had no talent for. Swimming was one of them. I found a great guy in Tom McCarthy.

Early on, I had Michael at the YMCA swimming, but because he couldn't complete the standard test to move him into the next level, he was stuck in a class that was for much younger kids. I didn't think this the best scenario for Michael and asked about private lessons, but none were offered. I called the Paul J. Lydon Aquatic Center, which wasn't far from my home, and was put in touch with Tom.

Tom was a handsome, tall, distinguished-looking man with a full head of gray hair that looked great on him! Tom was in his sixties, a school teacher and vice principal for a local middle school. Just by talking with him on the phone, I knew working with Tom one-on-one would be great for Michael.

In the pool, Tom maneuvered Michael's arms to help him make big, full arm sweeps, and since Michael kicked like a frog instead of using the proper kicking position, Tom manipulated his legs as well. He gave Michael verbal and visual cues as they swam together, Tom sometimes swimming ahead to encourage Michael to follow. He used props like noodles and barbells in the pool to help Michael swim better.

One day at the pool in 2008 stood out for me. The sun was shining, it was about sixty degrees, and the sky was blue with not a cloud in sight. I would love to have this weather all year round, keep the cold weather away.

Michael had his goggles on, and Tom had him hold a kickboard to practice his kicks. I enjoyed watching Michael in the water because he looked great and was always smiling. His left side wasn't as strong or coordinated as his right—side effects of the seizure. He did try his hardest and managed to stay afloat. After the kickboard, he rolled onto his back, holding a Styrofoam barbell. Tom guided him, constantly maneuvering his legs and arms to keep them in line and in correct form.

"Right, left, right, left," Tom called out as he helped Michael with the various strokes. Michael held onto the barbell, keeping his face in the water. Tom tapped his hand, letting Michael know that he had to make the stroke with that hand, whether it be his left or his right. They continually alternated arms. Michael practiced holding his breath underwater. He grabbed a red noodle to hold himself up and put his head in the water. I was so proud of him.

Now he was on his back again, and Tom was manipulating his legs to not kick like a frog. "Look up," Tom said. "Keep in your line and check the stripe on the ceiling."

Up and down the pool, again and again. Repetition, repetition, repetition. This was what will make Michael successful.

He made progress a little at a time, but it was progress none-theless. As he came close to me, sitting on the bench writing, I got the biggest smile from him ever. My day was complete.

I hated indoor pools. They smelled so strongly of chlorine, and the entire facility was always wet. The walls started out as a pretty blue but eventually muddled into an unappealing blue/brown/gray hue. It was also warm and clammy, like a sauna. I had to dress in layers, taking off clothes as time passed. When I left, I felt as if I'd had a smelly facial.

As awful as the pool looked and smelled, I have had some of my greatest moments here. Michael had come a long way. I was so happy that I decided to engage a swim instructor for him, and felt lucky to have found one in Tom. His patience, kindness and perseverance were truly what Michael needed. It was a blessing to watch, made better by the fact that I no longer had to be in the pool. Thanks to Tom, today Michael is a confident swimmer, he loves it so much.

Michael loved the end of the half-hour swim lesson because he got to dive for the rings, which gave him a feeling of great accomplishment. In the midst of the gray-blue walls and the drab atmosphere, he grabbed the brightly colored ring—red, green, orange—and broke the water's surface with the ring, some encouragement from us, and a huge smile.

Michael was also a big music lover. He played the trumpet in the school band and had private lessons with Mat Repucci.

He may not be the most gifted trumpet player, but music let him be a part of something, and he got a lot of enjoyment out of it. Matt, Michael's trumpet teacher, was also very patient with Michael and gave him all the extra clues he needed to play the trumpet successfully. Matt played trumpet in a local orchestra, and Michael and I attended all his concerts.

Michael's tutor, Katie Provost, has been coming to my house for six years. She was another blessing to us, and had the patience of Job. She helped Michael with reading, math, and any homework he may have that day. She was also helpful to me with reviewing his Individualized Education Plan (IEP) and helping me choose curriculums that best fitted Michael's learning style.

As I have learned over the years, it took many educated, patient, and caring people to help shape and mold a child like Michael. Michael has learned and grown so much, beyond anything I think the doctors thought he could accomplish. Daily I continued to try to see all the good Michael has accomplished, and not focus on what he can't do, hoping and praying for more, but resting in the moments of accomplishment that day.

> *Ask and it will be given to you: seek and you will find; knock and the door will be open to you.*
>
> *—Matthew 7:7*

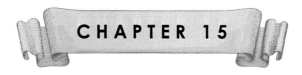

CHAPTER 15

Running and Friends: My Own Personal Saviors

DURING THE TWELVE YEARS OF dealing with Michael's cancer, running saved me. Being able to lace up my sneakers and go for a run anywhere, anytime was awesome! Just to escape the world, even if it was just for thirty minutes, was rewarding to me. My neighborhood was a great place to run through. Since it's a private development, the streets were safer to run in, even in the winter months when sidewalks sometimes weren't plowed. Running on the small side streets of the neighborhood was more intimate, safer than going on the roads more traveled. I ran down Old Haswell Park Road to Gallucia Road, to Tyler Lane, and up DeRosier hill, my usual route.

I often ran early in the morning, even though it was still dark. I took Boomer with me to keep me company. Boomer was happy to run with me, and made me feel safe. I would listen to my iPod and just think about my day, how it would unfold, who needed to be where, and how they would get there. As I ran, my thoughts often rambled. Once I had the thought, S*omeone in our neighborhood will get breast cancer.* This didn't alarm me, which may seem weird. It was just a random, fleeting thought, and I never really gave it much credence. It was just a thought, maybe prompted by something I had recently seen or read. I would carry on with my run.

During an uncharacteristic Saturday afternoon run in 2008, another random thought came to me: *Does Kaitlin's soccer coach carry a first aid kit?* Why would I think about that? Again, maybe I had seen one recently, who knew? I had no clue and continued on my run. As I ran toward the corner of my street, Old Haswell Park Road, I saw Mark in the car at the top of the street. *That is strange, why is he waiting for me?*

He rolled down his window and said, "Kaitlin got hit in the nose at her soccer game, the coach is bringing her to MGH. They think it may be broken." I jumped into the car, all sweaty, and Mark and I made our way to the MGH emergency room once again. As we drove, I told Mark about my random thought. He said, "That is weird." I agree!

Then I recalled the other thought I'd once had, the one about someone getting breast cancer in our neighborhood. Where were are all of these thoughts coming from? As we drove to MGH, I thought, *Is that God speaking to me?* No, I am just a typical person, nothing special, ordinary, why would God speak to me? I certainly don't deserve it, and I am no "holy person," like a priest or a nun. I brushed off the thought.

But it kept coming back, stronger, with the reminder that the twelve disciples were all ordinary, and God spoke to them. Yeah, but that was two thousand years ago; that doesn't happen today. But the more I tried to validate my reasoning, the more the thought recurred. "God is the same, yesterday, today, forever." Hebrews 13:8. I guess I retained and understood more than I thought as I read my Bible daily. Something was happening inside of me, but again I wasn't alarmed. I didn't understand fully what it was, but had an idea, and as we drove to MGH that day, I stopped pushing the thoughts away and instead rested in them.

After those early morning runs in the dark, once I was done, I would often just look up at the sky and stare at the stars. They were like diamonds sparkling so bright, as if they were all winking at me saying, "Yes, Jodi, we know what you are going through, and it will all be fine." I would take a deep breath, enjoying the quiet, then open the front door and start my day with my family.

My days started at 5:00 a.m. I made coffee and took it downstairs to my prayer room to pray with my prayer books to center myself, wake up, and clear my mind. I tried not to think about the day and what I had to accomplish. *Keep the slate clear and be still and listen.*

I prayed for everyone in my prayer book and anyone who asked me to pray for them. I put all their names in a notebook and lifted my notebook up to heaven and ask God to meet their needs. I prayed for my family, friends, and people who simply aggravated me, the ones who got under my skin and pushed my buttons. Those were the hardest to pray for. I read certain scriptures and meditated on them and how they related to my life and me. I tried to stay in my room for an hour each day, and then it was out the door for a run, or gym, or work or just being with family.

I liked my routine, and I was very glad I have a plan for myself. It kept me focused, motivated, and spiritually growing. Without all of that, I wouldn't be able to continue daily. My strength came from my deep faith, exercising, nutrition, family, and friends.

Friends. Nothing defines that word more than what I've seen in my friends in the past years. I got cards and letters and e-mails from so many friends who had heard about Michael's illness, and then mine. Many would just say *Thinking of you,* some would send prayers and encouragement, putting us on their prayer chains. Many were just acquaintances, people I had met over the years. Many were close friends. I enjoyed reading the cards and notes, and I felt the comfort and peace of their prayers.

My sister-in-law Pam was always sending cards and lip gloss and Avon stuff to Kaitlin and Jordan, helping them feel like not all the attention was on Michael. My friend, Deb, offered to pick Michael up one day a week after school so I could play tennis. She had two boys, and all three boys enjoyed their afternoon together.

One of my friends, Lori, was also very helpful. We met when Kaitlin and her daughter Lora were in preschool. Kaitlin was three, Lora was four. They were in different classrooms, but somehow found each other. They became close friends, and so did Lora and I. Even when we moved to Middleton, and they to Swampscott, about thirty miles apart, we all managed to remain friends.

Lora was the friend who would call and say, "I made dinner for you, and I am dropping it off at 2:00. Josh has skating at a local rink, so I'll be in the neighborhood." And sure enough, Lora would walk in with a smile, toting the most delicious dishes. One of our favorites was an acorn squash and bean stew, spicy and very flavorful. She was a good cook and would always choose healthy and nourishing dishes for us. She put the dish on the counter, gave me a hug and a kiss, chatted a bit, then took off to join Josh at the rink. She did this often. It could take an hour to get to my house, but Lora made the trip many times with food deliveries, or to collect Kaitlin for a weekend visit to their home. Kaitlin loved being with Lora and her family.

My neighbor and long-time friend Jean was truly amazing, not only for helping out with little stuff like picking Kaitlin up for school, but would call from the local grocery store to say, "I am at Market Basket. Can I bring you some groceries, milk, bread or eggs?" There was usually something I needed, but my standard answer was always, "No, we're good." (I was still working on allowing others to help.) No sooner did I hang up the phone when my doorbell would ring. There would be Jean with bags of groceries and other necessities, always with a little something extra thrown in.

Her husband, Joe, was a great friend too. I'd known Joe since I was twelve. We both grew up in Winthrop, and he played on my brother's Little League team. We became fast friends when Mark and I started dating. Joe and Mark were friends too. Joe and Jean moved to Middleton in 1995, and we followed in 1997. We were house hunting but had never really considered Middleton until I saw an ad in the newspaper about a new development being built. As it turned out, Wood Stone Estates abutted Joe and Jean's development, Bayberry Place. Mark and I went to view the property, deciding that it was a great location. Funny how things work out. How fortunate we were to have our two best friends so close by, and little did we know how much we would need them.

Mark traveled a lot, so through the years, Joe would often call me on his way home from work. "Just checking in on you," he'd say. Joe was easy to talk to, a practical, methodical thinker. I came to rely on him when Mark was out of town. Joe was a straight shooter, and I appreciated his honesty and compassion.

During one of Mark's business trips, Michael experienced a stroke-like seizure. Suddenly, he was unable to talk clearly, and the left side of his body became droopy. I called 911, and immediately Michael and I were being rushed to MGH by ambulance. I called Joe. He worked in Boston, and I knew he could easily get to MGH. He met us at the emergency room. It was such a relief to see his face. He gave me a hug. I was so grateful to have a friend with me. Michael was still unable to speak clearly or move the left side of his body. He was pretty lifeless.

Dr. Ebb was called and came down to examine Michael. He ordered a series of tests, and assured me he would get them back as quickly as possible and stay on top of this for me. As we waited for the test results, Michael fell asleep, and I sat there and read my Bible aloud to Joe. He believed in prayer and the power it holds. But he also shared with me there were times in the beginning of Michael's illness that I scared him when I would say things like, "Michael will be all right," or "He will survive to be four, five and six years old." This was at the beginning, when even the doctors didn't hold out much hope for Michael, giving him six months to live. Even when the MRI was read incorrectly and the doctors thought the cancer was growing, I said to Joe, "No, it's not."

He would look at me with the most compassionate big, brown eyes and say, "Jodi, please listen to the doctors." I believe he wanted to believe, like me, but at the same time, Joe is a very practical guy, and his faith at the time was not where mine was. He loved me and supported me, but sometimes he would have to take a deep breath to understand me. I think that what really scared Joe was not me, so much as the amount of faith I was exhibiting! Honestly, sometimes it scared me too! Through this journey with Michael though, Joe's faith has grown, and as I sit here reading Bible scriptures to Joe, I know he gets it and has a greater understanding than he once did, when I "scared him."

After several hours that day, the test came back, showing that Michael's Dilantin level was too low. They beefed it up with an IV, and soon Michael woke up more. He was talking normally and moving freely. Soon he was looking for something to eat. Amazing! Michael was back. What a relief! Joe and I hugged and cried tears of happiness. There were similar times that I called on Joe, and he was always there for me. Always willing to help, willing to drop whatever he was doing to help my family and me. Joe went to get the car, and Dr. Ebb escorted Michael and me out. As we drove home, I remember thinking, *God, you have put the most amazing people in my life. I could not do any of this without them!* Now content and happy, we made a quiet journey back to Old Haswell Park Road, to home.

-->)(*--

"Are you coming in to pray over me?" Those eight words are always the last words coming out of Michael's mouth each night. He helps to remind me about the importance of persistence. The night before this writing, however, was different.

Michael brushed his teeth and got ready for bed. I was ready for bed too so I climbed in my bed and got under my covers, waiting for Michael to finish up and hear him yell those eight words. He didn't.

Instead, he came in our room and said, "Mom, can I tuck you in?"

"Sure."

He climbed into bed next to me, put his head on my chest, then I heard those words: "Pray over me." I did, he kissed me, got me a glass of water, put it on my nightstand, and turned out the light. He went into his room and read for a little while. He talks out loud when he reads, so I could hear him.

As I lay there in bed, tucked in by my son, I couldn't help but think, *Yes, he will be all right. What the future holds for Michael only God knows, but I know it will be great!*

> *Jesus Christ is the same yesterday, today and forever!*
>
> —*Hebrews 13:8*

CHAPTER 16

Answered Prayers

MICHAEL WAS TWELVE IN 2008 and pretty good about knowing when his shunt wasn't working properly. He had three shunts in his head due to having hydrocephalus.

"I think my shunt is blocked," said Michael as we walked around Toys 'R Us on a busy Sunday before Christmas. That's the stuff that made my knees buckle underneath me, and my stomach felt like I could vomit on the spot.

But I was able to say, "Everything will be fine." I can't explain the peace that came over me when something like this happened. I didn't panic, I just prayed under my breath or in my mind, like the peace in the middle of the storm. This practice had become automatic, and let me function normally in this world.

Michael has had his shunts changed about twenty times. That meant twenty surgeries just for shunt revisions. He was an amazing kid.

We left the store, and Michael didn't speak a word in the fifteen-minute ride home. We pulled into the driveway and Michael said, "I can't move." Often Michael would say, "I can't move," or "My legs are broken." He'd had seizures before where the left side of his body goes "dead." He couldn't talk or move his left arm or leg, almost like a stroke.

My gut said and hoped that wasn't the case here, and I said, "I will meet you in the house." He eventually followed me in.

Both Michael and I could be stubborn, but I generally won. When it comes to Michael's illness though, sometimes it was a lot of wait and see.

He lay on the couch all that Sunday, and vomited about five times. All signs indicated that Michael was right, the shunt was not working. I sat next to him, read and prayed, and thought about how much I didn't like this and how I have had enough. Michael had his shunt repaired in June, just six months ago, and six months before that. For the past five years, it seemed that every six months required surgery for a blocked shunt.

Dr. Butler, the neurosurgeon, explained it to us, "It's because the fluid in Michael's head is thick and syrupy due to the cancer. It clogs the tubes that attempt to keep those fluids flowing."

Consequently, Michael sometimes experienced headaches ten times worse than a migraine. The good news was, once we had the shunt repaired, Michael bounced back pretty quickly.

That night, as we were lying on the sofa, Michael turned to me and asked, "Am I going to pass away, you know, die?"

I thought I was going to throw up. As I held back tears, I told him, "No, honey, it's just a plumbing problem. It can be fixed."

We'd been through this many times, and it would get fixed, and he'd be home in a few days. Michael was getting older and understanding his illness more and more. But since his grandfather, Stan, my father-in-law, had passed away, Michael was thinking more about being sick and dying. Stan's was really the first death that Michael had experienced. They were close too and talked frequently. Michael missed him very, very much.

Stan had been sick for years. He had heart valves replaced several times and, due to his illness, was on a lot of medication for a long time. He was a funny, tough kind of guy who always could light up a room. He often teased his nurses and doctors and say after surgery, "I can't move my legs," and get them all going, only for everyone to get a good laugh when they knew he was joking.

He often introduced himself as "Nunzio Fergone," or "Dudley Fafner," anything to get a chuckle. He fought the obstacles that his illness presented, along with my mother-in-law, Arlyne. What a great pair they made! They would still hug and kiss each other and walk hand in hand to all the doctor appointments and hospital visits. She took such great care of him for many years, all with the utmost love. Their marriage was a great blessing for me to see, such unconditional love, really what true love is all about. Stan died on September 11, 2008, twenty-six years to the day from when, Michael, Mark's older brother, had died.

When we came home that day and told Michael Grampie had died, he cried a bit, but was very quiet. The next day, he was down in the basement playing, and I peeked around the corner and noticed he was crying. I left him alone and gave him some time. A few minutes later, I came downstairs calling his name, so he knew I was on my way. I told him it was okay to cry and we are all sad. He didn't say much, just wanted to be left alone and seemed at that moment so grown up. Trying to be strong and brave, yet so real and emotional.

He attended the funeral and wake with us. I knew Michael was sad and upset and realized just how sad he was when he refused to bring up the gifts at mass. He just sat next to Mark and cried.

My son's first experience with death, an awful time, and there was no way for me to comfort him, no way for me to change how he was feeling.

After Michael spent that Sunday on the couch, the next morning, Mark, Michael, and I were off to MGH to see Dr. Butler. CT scans revealed fluid build-up—"hydrocephalus and a blocked shunt." Surgery was scheduled for later that day. The waiting began. Hopefully, he would be in by 6:00 tonight. We sat and waited, thought, prayed, read, and prayed some more.

We had been through this so many times, but it didn't get any easier for Michael or for us.

It was 10:00 at night when the transport team finally came to get Michael. I put his hospital Johnny on him. There were colorful stars all over them, one of God's great reminders to me. I smiled. Michael was transported to the OR, and Mark and I once again donned our Smurf-like, blue scrubs. It was hard to kiss him and leave him in the OR. He was brave and did very well, but it never got easier for me.

Mark and I had been at the hospital all day and were starving. One of the hardest things about waiting during a late-night surgery is that there was nothing to eat. So Mark and I didn't eat while waiting because Michael is starving and he wanted to eat too! But, of course, prior to surgery—no food allowed! We grabbed whatever was available, and then Mark headed home. He'd sleep at home with Kaitlin and make sure she was all set and had her homework all done We hugged and kissed good-bye at the elevator, and the door closed.

I was now comfortable staying with Michael; we'd been through this so much that it was routine. I walked the blue hallway with fish decals back to Michael's room. I climbed into Michael's bed and fell asleep.

We were waiting to hear from Dr. Butler, who had always referred to Michael as "the boy." At first, I was taken aback by his lack of sensitivity. He had known Michael for over ten years and had performed many surgeries. Shouldn't he know Michael's name by now? I just think neurosurgeons did this to avoid getting too attached. After all, they were opening up his head! I guess it really doesn't matter what Dr. Butler calls him, he was the best pediatric neurosurgeon in the world and took very good care of Michael. He can call him anything he wants. I had nothing but admiration and confidence in him.

That night, Dr. Butler came in about midnight, wearing his blue hospital scrubs.

"Everything is fine. We're just finishing up, and Michael will be moved to the PACU shortly."

I waited a few minutes then headed down to the second floor, where I'm buzzed in to the PACU after telling them that I am Michael's mom. Shortly after, a nurse with colorful hospital scrubs comes out to greet me, introducing herself as Michael's nurse. She looks familiar to me, and I to her.

"We have been here so many times, so I am sure we've met," I said to her.

When I got to Michael's bed, he was crying, "I want to go home."

It broke my heart. I wanted to crawl into bed with him and wrap my arms around him and take it all away. We finally got Michael to calm down and fully wake up. I gave him some ice chips. That was all he was allowed—no water, no nothing, we didn't want him to be sick from the anesthesia

Transport took us back to Ellison 17, where we both fell asleep and, thankfully, slept through the night, a major miracle with nurses coming in regularly to check Michael's vital signs, pumps beeping, and the dreaded flashlight test. Because Michael had neurosurgery, neurological tests had to be administered every two hours. They aimed a flashlight into his eyes and asked him to look up, look down, look left, look right. "What day is it?" "Do you know where you are?" "Who is the president?" "What is your name?"

One time, Michael didn't answer the question "What is your name?" He said he didn't know. The nurse freaked out! I sat up in the bed next to him and said, in my most stern voice, "Just tell the nurse your name so she can go away, and we can get back to sleep."

"Michael," he said.

We finally got back to sleep when it seemed like only minutes later the overhead lights flared on. It was like a Logan Airport runway in our room—so bright that you could land a plane in that room. Nuero rounds very early. It was 6:00 a.m.!

They were all wishing us a cheery good morning, but I was not even up or dressed. I jumped out of bed, with no bottoms on, and no one seemed to notice as I dressed in front of them.

Michael didn't respond to their questions and seemed lethargic. "We've only had a few hours sleep," I explained.

"We'll leave you alone for now, but we'll be coming up sometime today for a CT scan to make ensure that the new shunt is working properly," they told us.

By 10:00 a.m., when transport came to get Michael, he still hadn't eaten and seemed lethargic, just not his usual self. We left Ellison 17 for the CT scanner once again. As we trudge through the gray-green hallways, I donned my full metal jacket.

The technicians were always so funny, asking, "Is there a chance you could be pregnant?" I just laughed, as it would have to have been an immaculate conception! I stood next to Michael as they strapped him into the scanner and placed his head in the tube. His eyes were closed, and he just didn't seem good to me.

The scan took only a few minutes, and before we knew it we were back on Ellison 17. Dr. Butler's team arrived shortly after to explain that the right side of his shunt is cleared, but the left side was blocked. Sometimes when Dr. Butler repaired the right side, which communicated with the left side, it would unblock the left side too. Dr. Butler always tried to do the least invasive surgery on Michael and not to have his head open too long, which could lead to further complications. All in all, Michael was to have twenty different shunt surgeries; this was just one of many.

Dr. Butler's attending physician, Elizabeth Shannon, came in. Frankly, she was a lot more personable that Dr. Butler. Friendly, with a more happy-go-lucky personality, pretty, blond, and about forty years old. She wore purple scrubs and a heavily starched white lab coat with handwritten note pads in her coat pockets.

She pulled up a chair next to me and leaned over with her hands on her lap. She looked me right in the eye and said, "Mom, Dr. Butler wants Michael to have another surgery today. He was hoping that the one surgery would unblock both sides, but it wasn't successful. We're waiting to hear from the OR as to when it will take place, but it will be sometime today."

I nodded numbly. Elizabeth was always so reassuring.

"We want Michael feeling his usual self and we know this is not it, so we'll do everything to get him into surgery as quick as possible, so he can get better." After that, she left to make sure Michael had a spot in the OR that day. Elizabeth was feisty, pushy, and I counted on her to "move things along," always keeping Michael's best interests at heart. She was always giving me her card, saying "If you need anything, or if they don't come to get Michael for his head scan in one hour, have me paged." She was the best at getting things done, and I loved having her on Michael's team!

So we waited, prayed, thought, waited, and prayed some more. Michael was clearly not feeling well and just slept. I couldn't concentrate on the television, or think about anything but Michael. I didn't want to have to go through another surgery.

I looked down at my New Balance gym bag and saw my sneakers—my 768 Carolina Blue with a touch of lipstick pink. My sneakers had always served me well, and I suddenly couldn't sit any longer. I needed to run. I donned my running gear, and as I bent down to lace up my sneakers, I thought, *How happy I am to have you, my sneakers!*—sneakers that gave me the strength to walk out of this hospital, even for a short time.

I found Michael's nurse. "I've going to take a run. I'll be back in thirty minutes," I told her.

"No problem," she assured me. "I'll check in on him while you're gone." Michael's team of nurses was great, and I felt blessed to have them.

As I headed to the elevators, I felt better already, to have the ability to run along the Charles River, listen to my iPod and temporarily leave it all behind me. I knew everything at the hospital would be there, waiting for me, nothing different, nothing changed when I got back, but *I* would be different! I would have let it go by looking at the beauty of the day, the water, the people, the sky, breathing in the air, sweating, and being part of the world I love. Lose my breath, huff and puff, and feel accomplished, if only for thirty minutes. Before I knew it, I walked back into MGH through the turnstiles again, but with a little more spring in my step, a clearer and more confident *me! Michael and I will get through this. I just know it.*

Michael wasn't complaining, but he was listless and sleepy, and really didn't feel well. The nuero team came to get Michael at 2:00 to take him to the operating room. I donned the ridiculous Smurf outfit once again, and walked into the operating room as Michael was wheeled on the stretcher. After a short wait, he was given his cocktail of Propofol. After one big yawn, his eyes rolled back, and he was asleep.

I got escorted to the exit, but not before I removed my lovely outfit. The doors opened, and I stood in the hall waiting for the elevator to take me back to Ellison 17 and more waiting. I just wanted to go home, as Michael had expressed after his surgery yesterday. I wasn't anxious or scared, just exhausted.

In Michael's room, I took a much-needed shower. The showers at MGH reminded me of what showers must be like in prison—cold, not much water pressure, and soap that dried the heck out of your skin and didn't smell very good. The towels were so rough it was like toweling yourself off with sandpaper. I got dressed and lay down on Michael's bed to wait.

Again.

I was awakened by Dr. Butler saying, "Everything went well."

I made my way down to the PACU and rang the buzzer. The nurse recognized me, and we laughed.

"Yes, I was here yesterday."

This time, as I approached Michael, I could tell he was better. No crying and he looked himself. Shortly, we were wheeled back to Ellison 17. Already I can see Michael improving; he was much more alert, and hungry, good signs. We had a CT scan scheduled for tomorrow to make sure all the shunts were clear and working and if, all goes well, we could go home tomorrow.

Since Mark was away working, I called my parents to let them know what was going on. They would come in tomorrow and take Michael and I home.

I've already got one foot out the door. Michael was looking good, and I never wanted to stay here any longer than I had to. I planned on Michael recovering and doing all the things he needed to do to be released and get us out of here—walk, eat, and pee!

He usually bounced back pretty quickly, so I felt safe in assuming that tomorrow we'd be going home. For the remainder of the day, Michael ate, walked, and peed. We had the CT scan, and all of the shunts were clear. We'd be leaving tomorrow.

The next day, Pauline and Frank, my parents, came to take us home. My parents were the best, the most accommodating and available people I know. No matter what I needed, they were there, for their family and for others. Whether it was a financial need, someone to talk to, a shoulder to cry on, babysitting, or child-rearing advice, you name it, they delivered. They always have and still do. I often forgot that they are in their late seventies because they just didn't seem old.

They were thrilled to be able to take Michael and me home. They drove from Winthrop to MGH, then took us back to Middleton. My mom picked up lunch for all of us to have when we got home, and cooked dinner for us that night. I couldn't ask for more. All is done with love and compassion.

Jean, my neighbor friend, stopped by and dropped off Kaitlin as Kaitlin had stayed at her house the night before. Jean came complete with groceries and flowers! As we all settled back into our home, I looked around my house, at my parents, Kaitlin, Michael, Boomer, my couch, my bed, my bathroom, my shower, my towels. I felt blessed to be home! I couldn't think of any place else I would rather be.

It had been ten years since Michael was diagnosed and back in 1998, I had thought that Michael's illness would be a very small chapter of our life. But ten years later, I realized that it wasn't just a chapter of our lives, it was the book.

And yet, I really couldn't complain.

-➤➤❦❦-

On a cold November day, it was raining out and I'd just gotten home from work. *I'll hit the bathroom then head down to the bus stop to get Michael so he doesn't walk home in the rain.*

As I walked downstairs, I looked out the window and saw the bus up the street, early. There was Michael with his hands in his pockets, backpack on, walking toward the house with the biggest smile on his face.

At the front door, I said, "Sorry, I wanted to get you so you didn't have to walk in the rain."

"That's okay." He gave me a big kiss and walked into the house. That was one of my best days! The little things, the day-to-day things, that defined a great life. Michael taught me that lesson, and he'll continue to teach me so much! He gave me many aha moments that took my breath away.

Due to the initial seizure in 1998 from to the stem cell transplant, Michael was developmentally delayed. He was on an Individual Education Plan (IEP) at school, and attended a separate classroom at Howe Manning Middle School for most of his instruction. He took the regular bus to school. Being on an IEP meant school open houses were different. Even though he started every day in the same homeroom as all the other sixth graders, his curriculum was very different. So we always went to the "small" classroom for our open house.

Open house to me was a slap in the face, a punch in the stomach. There were no papers in the hall with Michael's name, no drawings on the bulletin boards, no awards for scholastic achievement. Open houses always made me realize where Michael should be in reading, writing, and math, and I knew in my heart how far behind he was compared to other sixth graders. Actually, anything that involved Michael took on a different meaning. Baseball tryouts were always difficult. Michael realized his limitations and became intimidated by the other kids. He was in Little League by this time, but next year he would actually have to try out for a team, which probably meant the end of baseball for Michael.

Even though baseball probably wouldn't be long in Michael's future, I wanted to give him the confidence to continue with it as long as he could. Since Peter, my trainer, was so helpful to me, I decided to have Michael train with him.

I was surprised at how well Michael took to Peter, and Peter to Michael. Peter was well-built, of course, with thick, dark hair, and expressive brown eyes. With his dark complexion and great smile, Michael was at ease with him right away.

I explained to Peter about Michael's limitations, but he wasn't fazed by it at all. Peter trained professional athletes, your average guy and gal, and other children with disabilities. He treated them all the same. His most common after-workout comment was "He did what he was capable of for the hour. It was a successful session."

Michael wanted to play baseball but had a hard time with coordination; he couldn't catch the ball. Peter worked with him on those skills at a local racquetball court.

As I watched them one day, Michael painfully missed catching eight balls, then nine, then ten. It was very hard to watch him miss time and time again. As he missed, my own body lunged forward, toss after toss, as if I can could catch them for him. Michael was twelve; he should be able to catch a ball!

Finally he caught one, and I cried. I'd never thought that such simple things would be so difficult for Michael; I just didn't know what to expect. He caught another ball and another, and my tears turned to smiles. All he needed was enough repetition, and he'd get it.

Now Michael was hitting the balls with the racket. They went everywhere, of course, bouncing off the walls, but he was having fun, and in the racquetball court, you always looked successful—it just had to bounce off the walls. Again, it took him many tries to hit the ball.

"Watch the ball, watch the ball," Peter coached him with another throw to Michael.

He swung and missed, again and again and again. Then he hit one.

What a great feeling for Peter, for him, for me!

Peter was one-of-a-kind, and practiced himself what he preached to others. He led with his heart, and treated his clients as if they were his only client. He was totally focused on you for that hour, and beyond. Often he'd said to me, "I train the hardest muscle, the one in the center of your body: your heart. If you can get someone to feel the motivation and inspiration in their heart as you train them, the success will come." What Michael and I learned in an hour training session with Peter carried with us beyond the walls of the gym.

Michael's team consisted of not only trainers, but teachers, a great group of educators—a homeroom teacher, a special education teacher, a personal aide, an occupational therapist, a physical therapist, a speech therapist, a psychologist and band, art, computer, library, and gym teachers. They were the foundation of a terrific support system that kept Michael's best interests at heart. They kept me updated with all his progress and sent home things for him to practice on his own.

In April 2008, we had an IEP meeting, one that again reinforced for me that Michael would always be behind his peers. The room was small and cramped, and the table so small that we all couldn't fit around it. In addition to Mark and me, Michael's special needs teacher, regular classroom teacher, school psychologist, occupational therapist, physical therapist, speech therapist, and nurse were all present. The room was hot to me. With no air, I felt almost suffocated.

We all signed in. "Do you have any specific concerns?" we asked.

"No, no, we'll just ask questions as we go along."

If Michael had any testing done over the past year, all his test scores were read back to us (in addition to a written report we'd received before). This was done so everyone on the team had a sense of Michael's progress:

Verbal comprehension 67, extremely low.

Perceptual Reasoning 61 extremely low.

Working Memory 50 extremely low.

Processing Speed 50 extremely low.

Full scale 49 extremely low.

Listening comprehension 64, extremely low.

Word recognition 40, extremely low.

Math problem solving 46, extremely low.

Numerical operations 49, again extremely low.

All extremely low.

As they read off his scores, I was getting hotter and hotter. Tears welled up in my eyes, my heart was in my throat, and my ears began to hum. My shoulders tightened and lifted up; they were almost touching my ears. The tension in my body was as high as it could; my body was as stiff as a board.

I knew all the results, I'd read them and know what they mean. But sitting there and listening to "extremely low" time and time again was enormously difficult. I held back my tears. "Can you give me an example of how Michael was tested on working memory?" I asked, trying to understand.

"We asked him to repeat a sentence word for word. For example, 'John was told by his teacher Mrs. Jones to go into the classroom and get his notebook binder and backpack.' He should have repeated the sentence back exactly, but his response was 'The teacher told the kid to get his notebook, binder, and backpack.'"

That response gets Michael no points and a low score. I laughed because Michael got the concept, and I already knew his memory was impaired from the brain tumor. So for me, standard tests weren't beneficial, but they helped the teachers and school assess him against his peers and got him all the help he needed. I knew that was good in actuality, but it still made me frustrated and mad. We already knew that he would always come up very short when stacked up against children his age. These meetings were a painful—and concrete—reminder.

Each teacher read Michael's previous goals to us, and then they let us know if Michael had reached those goals. As a team, they then set up new goals for Michael's next school year.

The teachers tried to be kind to us and always started their reports with positives. "Michael is a pleasure to work with." "Michael tries so hard when he is with me." "I know Michael will be successful in life; he has such a great attitude." "I wish all my students were are conscientious as Michael." "Michael's face and smile makes my day." All things they truly meant and felt. This part always made me cry too, but joyful tears at this point.

Michael did improve slowly each year, but not fast enough for me.

An Individual Education Plan review comprised two meetings of two to three hours each. We reviewed his progress for the year—where he was and where they thought he'd be at this time next year. It was always heart-wrenching. In addition to the IEP, we also reviewed neuropsych exams, which were never a happy report. I always left feeling drained and unsure.

Although I knew in my heart that God had a plan—a great plan—some days it was harder to believe than others. Those days of IEP meeting days, or attending a baseball game where Michael swung and missed almost every ball pitched to him, those were days when it was much harder to believe in God's plan.

After one of those grueling IEP meetings in 2009, I was in my kitchen, putting away the dishes. I glanced out the window and saw the neighborhood kids playing basketball. Michael was their age, and he should have been out there playing too. Instead he was in the house, playing Legos or a video game. He couldn't keep up with kids his own age, socially and physically. Many times I made him go out and play with the other kids, but just ten minutes later, he was back. "I am done playing," he'd say.

That was hard for me, mostly because I thought about how I would feel, not having many friends and not being involved in the neighborhood activities. But the truth was, Michael didn't care. He was content doing his own thing. He did have a few friends at school and seemed to be happy with just the few.

I asked myself, *What is the one thing I wish for all my kids?* The answer has always been, *For them to be happy.*

I asked myself, *Do you think Michael is happy? Yes, he was the happiest kid I know, always in a good mood.*

I stopped looking out the window and continued to put the dishes away. Just another day in the journey. I moved on and let it go. I thanked God that there are only twenty-four hours in a day. After an IEP meeting, I usually got home and prayed, thanking God for all that Michael could do. I'd go to bed, knowing that tomorrow was a new beginning.

Each night I open my Bible, I take comfort in the words, noticing the passage of time shown in its worn pages, the watermarks from my tears, a coffee stain here, pink highlighter there. There are notes, cards, yellow legal paper stuffed in between the pages, a constant reminder of the many people who have touched—and blessed—my life. I read the passage:

"Jesus said to him, "If you can! Everything is possible to one who has faith" (Mark 9:23).

I know tomorrow will be better, filled with hope, faith, desire, expectations, and endless possibilities.